WX 153 WID

THE WIDENING GAP

Health inequalities and policy in Britain

Mary Shaw, Daniel Dorling, David Gordon
and George Davey Smith

First

D0573977

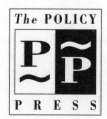

The POLICY
P~P
PRESS

FIRST UNITED NATIONS DECADE FOR THE
eradication of poverty
(1997-2006)

First published in Great Britain in November 1999 by

The Policy Press
University of Bristol
34 Tyndall's Park Road
Bristol BS8 1PY
UK

Tel   +44 (0)117 954 6800
Fax   +44 (0)117 973 7308
E-mail tpp@bristol.ac.uk
http://www.bristol.ac.uk/Publications/TPP

ISBN 1 86134 142 3

Mary Shaw is a Research Fellow in the School of Geographical Sciences, **Daniel Dorling** is a Reader and Fellow in the School of Geographical Sciences, **David Gordon** is Head of the Centre for the Study of Social Exclusion and Social Justice, School for Policy Studies and **George Davey Smith** is Professor of Clinical Epidemiology, Department of Social Medicine, all at the University of Bristol.

Photograph on front cover kindly supplied by Mary Shaw.

Cover design by Qube Design Associates, Bristol.
Printed in Great Britain by Hobbs the Printers Ltd, Southampton.

Contents

List of tables and figures

Tables

Figures

Foreword

Peter Townsend

This book makes the case for re-invigorating the political priority afforded to health inequalities in Britain by demonstrating unequivocally how the contemporary health divide my colleagues and I identified over two decades ago has continued to widen since that time. The book takes our early work forward in a number of ways. At the simplest level it updates our statistics, but it also updates our methods, our understanding of the processes involved and refines the policy options we presented two decades ago with both hindsight and insight. What this book calls for is a rethinking of government policy on inequalities in health. The book's authors are kind enough to start their study by referring to the Black Report and so I too will start there in my explanation of why we need changes in policy in order to reduce inequalities in health in Britain today (for a fuller version of the arguments see 'Structural plan needed to reduce inequalities of health' in the companion volume to this book – *Inequalities in health: The evidence* (edited by Gordon et al, 1999).

The Black Report of 1977-80 (DHSS, 1980; Townsend and Davidson, 1988; see Glossary) showed that inequalities in health had been widening since the 1950s, that this trend was principally related to inequalities of material resources, and that a programme of higher social security benefits and more equal distribution of income, as well as action on housing and services, was required. The Report was rejected by the Conservative government at the time of its publication, principally on the grounds of cost. Yet the Report continued to exert influence on research and over the next two decades that research continued to point to the need for structural action to achieve better health among the population of Britain. For example, a report for the Health Education Council in 1987 listed hundreds more papers with new research evidence generally supporting this position; the same position being advocated by this book (Whitehead, 1987; and see Townsend and Davidson, 1988).

After winning the election of May 1997 the Labour government set up an Independent Inquiry to examine inequalities in health. This reported in December 1998 (*Independent Inquiry into Inequalities in Health*, 1998). The central thrust of the Inquiry's recommendations reflected those put forward in the Black Report. The Inquiry's report demonstrated the heightened health problems created by dramatically widening living standards since the late 1970s. There were 39 principal recommendations. The all-important one was No 3, which specified the need for policies to "reduce income inequalities and improve the living standards of households in receipt of social security benefits" (*Independent Inquiry into Inequalities in Health*, 1998, p 36). Benefits in cash or in kind had to be increased to reduce "poverty in women of childbearing age, expectant mothers, young children and older people." The last chapter of this book expands on how this aim might be achieved.

Although the Independent Inquiry's report was extensive, it was at times unfocused. Some commentators fastened onto particular recommendations which, though important, are not central. Because there seemed to be some danger of the central thrust being missed, the original members of the 1977-80 Black Committee issued a report in March 1999 calling for a government plan to phase in better benefits for health (Black et al, 1999). This book provides further evidence of the need for that plan, partly by updating the Independent Inquiry's report, and partly by showing in greater detail how many people would suffer if inequalities in health are not reduced, and by clearly exposing the processes that are at work in producing these inequalities.

The White Paper of July 1999 *Saving lives: Our healthier nation* (DoH, 1999a) was the government's response to the Independent Inquiry. The White Paper made almost no mention of the growing inequality in income and of measures to boost the inadequate incomes of the poor, other than a reference to the Minimum Wage, to the Working Families Tax Credit and to the Childcare Tax Credit (DoH, 1999a, p 45). The government's initiatives on cancer, heart disease, accidents and mental illness were welcome, as was its acceptance that "while the roots of health inequality run deep, we refuse to accept such inequality as inevitable" (DoH, 1999a, p 44). However, the key message about the substantial structural action required in order to turn around the growing divisions in society, especially by addressing the inadequacy of many current social security benefits, was not raised or discussed. This is a further indication of why independent research, such as that presented here, is so badly needed.

Did the action report *Reducing health inequalities* (DoH, 1999c) also released in 1999 from the DoH, take up this missing theme? It described progress in addressing all 39 of the Independent Inquiry's recommendations. On the key recommendation – No 3 – attention was called to the government's commitment to tackling worklessness, including the New Deals for employment and tax and benefit reforms to "make sure that work pays, reform of the employer's contribution to help remove barriers to employment, and policies to improve skills through education and training." The report continued: "But we recognise the need to provide security for those who cannot work" (DoH, 1999c, p 6). There is no discussion of the exact meaning of security, or of minimally adequate standards of income for families with children, lone parents, disabled people and pensioners. The measures the government have taken (as quoted in the DoH action report) are listed in the box opposite.

There is no doubt that the 1997 Labour government is giving greater priority than did the preceding governments of the 1980s and 1990s to inequalities in health. Equally, there is no doubt that a range of measures, including many which are external to healthcare policy, are now in play. This is welcome. But serious questions need to be raised: (i) of the scale of action so far, (ii) of the effective management of the distribution of earnings and of disposable income, (iii) of the adequacy of income and of living standards generally of the many millions of people with no prospect of having paid employment. The new evidence presented in this book suggests that action has been too limited, that redistribution has not been addressed, and that poverty levels in Britain are far too high for us to expect to see inequalities in health fall.

Many of the recommendations made at the time of the Black Report have still to be addressed by the government even though their validity was underpinned by the 1998 Independent Inquiry's report and is reinforced even more robustly here. However, one very important recommendation from the Black Report has been adopted, at least in theory. To quote from the report:

> "We have tried to confine ourselves to matters which are practicable now, in political, economic and administrative terms, and which will, nonetheless, properly maintained, exert a long-term structural effect.... We have continued to feel it right to give priority to young children and mothers, disabled people and measures concerned with prevention.... Above all the *abolition of child poverty should be adopted as a national goal*.... (DHSS, 1980, p 195; my emphasis)

Reproduced in Table 1 are the principal recommendations made in the Black Report, with estimates of cost made at the time by the previous government, updated by the Department of Health to 1998. This table illustrates the kind of things the government would have to do to begin to achieve its aims. The specifics of many of these policies are outlined in Chapter 5 of this book.

Families with children

- An increase of £4.70 a week from October 1999 in the child premium in the income-related benefits (IRBs) for children under 11.

- Additional increases from April 2000 in the family and child premiums in the IRBs to match increases in Child Benefit.

Disabled people

- Extra help for young people disabled early in life: reform of Severe Disablement Allowance (SDA) to give people who are disabled and claim benefit before the age of 20 access to a higher rate of benefit than they would get from SDA and Income Support. The age limit is extended to 25 for those in higher education and vocational training whose course began before they were 20.

- Extra help for severely disabled people with the greatest care needs and the lowest incomes: Disability Income Guarantee will provide extra help in IRBs for people who receive the highest rate care component of Disability Living Allowance (DLA).

Pensioners

- A new Minimum Income Guarantee (at least £75 a week for single pensioners; £116.60 for a couple). This will make the poorest pensioners at least £160 a year better off in real terms from April 1999.

- The Minimum Income Guarantee will be uprated relative to earnings in April 2000 so that single pensioners will be an estimated £250 a year better off than in April 1998.

- A fivefold increase in the winter fuel payment and a new, more generous, Home Efficiency Scheme.

Source: DoH action report (1999)

Table 1: Annual cost of meeting the principal recommendations of the Black Report on inequalities in health, as estimated in 1982 and in 1996 prices

No.	Recommendation	£m 1982 prices (1)	£m 1996 prices (2)
10	Free milk for under-5s	300	700
12	Expansion of day care for under-5s	550*	1,250
23	Special programmes in 10 areas with highest mortality	65	50
24	Child Benefit increased to 5.5% of average gross male earnings	950+	2,200
25	Age-related Child Benefit	1,275‡	2,900
26	Maternity grant increased to £100	60	140
27	Infant care allowance	440§	1,000
28	Free school meals for all children (net extra cost)	640μ	1,460
29	Comprehensive disablement allowance	1,175¶	2,700
	Total annual cost	5,455	12,500
	Total cost (as % GDP)	2.2	1.7
	Total cost (as % social security)	13	11.7

Notes: * An initial capital cost of possibly £300-£400m would also be required.

+ Cost of raising Child Benefit to £7.57 per week.

‡ Assuming average increase of £3 per week for children aged 5-15.

§ The cost of a £5.85 per week benefit if half the 2.9 million women at home looking after children had a child under 5.

μ Assuming 70% take-up.

¶ As estimated by the Disability Alliance in 1981.

Source: (1) *Hansard* 16 December 1982, cols 242-3, reply by Kenneth Clarke MP to Gwynneth Dunwoody MP; (2) Reply by Tessa Jowell, Minister of State for Public Health, to a Parliamentary Question from Jean Corston MP 25 November 1998

History shows that governments can introduce radical changes but that when they occur they are ordinarily built on precedents and are divided into a succession of steps. To be influential, scientific advice has to be pitched in a practicable and manageable, as well as desirable, form. What matters first is for the government to change the direction of trends making for increased poverty and inequality. This depends on mobilising popular support for a number of principled measures, and introducing new institutions at the same time as strengthening existing ones. There exists overwhelming evidence of support, in a series of representative and reliable opinion polls, for the kind of measures listed in Table 1 (Jowell, 1991-98; see also Chapter 5). As the table shows, significant advances could be made with under 2% of GDP, or about a tenth of the current expenditure on social security – even if further steps need to be considered after five or ten years. The total amount is of an order illustrated by the Chancellor's decisions in 1997-98 to introduce the windfall tax (which should generate £5bn between 1997 and 2002), and to change tax allowances and National Insurance Contributions. Another indicator is the surplus of £2.5bn of contributions over payments in the National Insurance Fund in 1997-98, rising to £7bn a year in the following two years.

The task ahead, to reverse the widening of the health gap shown in Chapter 4 of this book, is daunting but must be accepted. One problem, which has not been examined by successive governments in the last two decades, is the effect of specific past and present policies on trends in the inequalities of living standards and hence health. The nearest attempt to doing this was in a report for the Joseph Rowntree Foundation (Hills, 1995; and see also Hills, 1998). The major influences need to be identified and explained. In Britain the policies producing increasing inequalities over the past two decades include (i) the abolition of the link between social security benefits and earnings, (ii) the restraints on the value of Child Benefit, (iii) the abolition of lone parent allowances and of the earnings-related addition to incapacity benefit, which allowed people disabled before pensionable age to draw early on their entitlement to the State Earnings Related Pension Scheme (SERPS), and (iv) the substitution of means-tested benefits for universal social insurance and for non-contributory benefits for particular population categories such as pensioners and disabled people.

What would be required to restore the UK to the much reduced range of inequality experienced 20 years ago? If the Conservative government had not reduced social security benefits, it can be estimated that the poorest 20% of the population would today have about £5bn, or 20%, more in aggregate disposable income, that the ratio between the richest and poorest 20% would be reduced from about 9:1 or 10:1 to 5:1, and that poverty by European standards would have been reduced by more than a third. Instead the UK has experienced the most severe growth of social inequality and of poverty, especially child poverty, of any European country. If you compare the inequality described in Chapter 2 of this book with that at the time of the original Black Report, the worsening of the situation is staggering.

In the 1998 budget statement the Chancellor announced a welcome increase in the rate of Child Benefit, together with improvements in Income Support rates for children. However, the increase applies only to the eldest child in the family and, since the real value of Child Benefit had fallen in previous years, the increase primarily represents a catching-up exercise. If the Chancellor also decides to tax the benefit, which has been suggested but for which there is little rational support (Clarke and McCrae, 1998; Dilnot 1998; Bradshaw, 1998; Bradshaw and Barnes, 1999: forthcoming), benefit may be withdrawn altogether from higher earning households at a later stage, and be converted into a means-tested benefit. In 1999 the government will also replace Family Credit with Working Families Tax Credit, which is designed to increase the level of benefit as well as the numbers entitled to it. This is also a means-tested scheme, intended to raise the numbers of low-earning families receiving such a tax credit by 400,000. On the basis of written answers to Parliamentary Questions (for example, *Hansard*, 28 July 1998, cols 188-90) and investigations on the minimum necessary family income, some experts have concluded after protracted research that the new credit "will not provide Low Cost Allowance level incomes to two-parent families"(Parker, 1998, p 88). On all the available evidence, means-tested benefits are poor in coverage, costly to administer, do not encourage savings, and are generally inadequate in meeting need, in addition to being highly unpopular.

As Chapter 3 of this book clearly demonstrates, the root cause of inequalities in health is poverty. The problem of poverty is larger than is often represented – there are numerous independent reports showing this (see for example, Cohen et al, 1992; NCH Action for Children, 1995,1998; Kempson, 1996; Gordon and Pantazis, 1997; Bradshaw, 1998). However, even narrowly drawn government statistics, for example, the annual Department of Social Security reports on *Households Below Average Income* (HBAI) (DSS, 1998a), reveal a serious divergence of living standards in the 1980s and 1990s. The number of adults and children with incomes below the low income standards set for 1979 has remained as high as, or even higher than, in 1979 itself (see Table 2). Thus, the latest HBAI report shows that there were 1.2 million children living on below half average 1979 household income after housing costs in 1979 but, despite a big increase in average national living standards especially for the rich in the intervening 17 years, there were 1.3 million children below that same absolute 1979 standard in 1996-97 (DSS, 1998a, p 229). If we look at the 'relative' situation in both 1979 and 1996-97 then the number of children in households with below half the average household income grew sharply from 1.2 million to 3.9 million.

The latest data show that the problem of poverty is still growing. Recent national survey data from the Office for National Statistics (ONS) show that the poorest 20% of households (nearly 12 million people), who depend on benefits for 80% of their income, had an average disposable weekly income of only £86 a week (at 1997-98 prices) in the financial year 1994-95 and, three years later, £87. The richest 20% of households had an average of £707 in 1994-95 which had advanced to £753 by 1997-98. The richest 20% had 8.2 times the income of the poorest 20% in 1994-95 and 8.6 times their income in 1997-98 (ONS, 1998a, Table 8.3). At the end of the 1990s the widening of disposable income is still continuing.

Table 2: **Number in population living below the government's two 1979 standards of low income, and below half contemporary average household income, excluding self-employed (millions)**

Standard	1979	1993-94	1994-95	1995-96
Below 1979 median income of lowest decile	2.8	3.0	2.9	3.0
Below half 1979 average household income	4.5 (children 1.2m)	4.35	4.25	4.4 (children 1.3m)
Below half contemporary average household income	4.5 (children 1.2m)	11.6	12.1	12.2 (children 3.9m)

Note: The data are adjusted according to the retail price index for the years in question. The corresponding totals, including the self-employed, are not given for these years, although they were given in earlier HBAI reports. These tended to show that the number of self-employed with incomes smaller than the two measures of low income had increased much faster than the number of employed.

Sources: DSS (1996, pp 226 and 229; 1997, pp 234 and 237; and 1998a, pp 227, 229 and 231)

With support from evidence such as that presented in this book the harmful effects on the distribution of income of particular policies – such as the abandonment of the link between earnings and benefits, cuts or reductions in benefits for some vulnerable groups and the flagging level of Child Benefit – have to be identified as obstacles to the reduction of inequalities in health. It is absolutely and fundamentally necessary for the government to implement fiscal policies which reverse the process of widening income inequality. That should be their top priority.

Acknowledgements

We acknowledge Crown Copyright for Census data; the Office for National Statistics (ONS) and General Register Office (Scotland) for mortality data; MORI and Domino films for the *Breadline Britain* data and Social and Community Planning Research (SCPR), London, for British Social Attitudes data.

We would like to acknowledge funding for George Davey Smith (GDS), Danny Dorling (DD) and Mary Shaw (MS) provided via the ESRC Health Variations Programme under the following grants: *Housing wealth and community wealth* (DD and MS) (L128251009); *Social position and health in ethnic communities* (GDS) (L128251007); *Stress, life-style and inequalities in ill-health* (GDS) (L128251037). Danny Dorling acknowledges ESRC grants for the following research: *Study of the 1997 general election* (H304253001) and *Providing local context for the 1997 general election* (R000222649). Mary Shaw is funded by an ESRC Fellowship (R000271045).

The authors would also like to acknowledge the funding support of the Joseph Rowntree Foundation for the projects: *Death in Britain* (DD) and *Inequalities in life and death* (DD and MS).

The authors would like to thank the following people for their support in producing this book: Lin Hattersley at the ONS for results derived from analyses of Longitudinal Study mortality data. Ron Johnston, Iain MacAllister, Charles Pattie, Bethan Thomas and Helena Tunstall for providing data. Simon Godden for the wonderful maps and Dave Worth for the layout. Helen Anderson, Jane Ferrie, Katherine French, Ron Johnston, Richard Mitchell, Nichola Tooke and Helena Tunstall for ploughing through drafts of various states of (in)completion. Liz Humphries for help with manuscript preparation. The three anonymous referees for their valuable comments. Peter Townsend for his suggestions and support. Finally, we would like to thank Dawn Pudney, our patient editor at The Policy Press.

Glossary

Black Report
The Black Report was commissioned at the end of the 1970s by the-then Labour government who appointed Sir Douglas Black to chair a working group to review the evidence on inequalities in health and to suggest policy recommendations that should follow. The original report was published (DHSS, 1980), although it was not widely available as only 260 copies were initially printed. The authors of the report were Sir Douglas Black, Professor J.N. Morris, Dr Cyril Smith and Professor Peter Townsend. A subsequent edition published by Penguin made the findings widely available and it was later published by Penguin in a dual volume together with Whitehead's *The health divide* (1987), which updated the findings. This version was edited by Peter Townsend and Nick Davidson, and it is this version of the report that we cite (Townsend and Davidson, 1988) as it is most widely available.

Constituency/Parliamentary constituency
An area used to elect Members of Parliament, made up of roughly 16 wards on average, each constituency has an average population of 74,000 people aged under 65. (*Source*: authors)

Correlation coefficient
A measure of the linear association between two variables (A and B). The correlation coefficient r can vary between -1 and +1. When r equals +1 there is a perfect positive linear relationship – as A rises, B rises proportionately. When r equals -1 there is a perfect negative linear relationship – as A rises, B falls proportionately. The size of the correlation coefficient between 0 and +/-1 indicates how close the association between the variables is. (*Source*: authors)

Death rate
An estimate of the proportion of a population that dies during a specified period. The number of persons dying during the period is divided by the number of persons in the population. This is then multiplied by

1,000, to give the death rate per 1,000. Rates can also be calculated per 10,000, 100,000 or per 1,000,000. (*Source*: adapted from Last, 1995)

Death rate ratio
This is the ratio of the death rate for one group compared to the death rate of another group. For example, if group A has a death rate of 8.4 per 1,000 and group B has a death rate of 4.2 per 1,000, the death rate ratio is 2:1. This is similar to the relative rate or relative risk of death. (*Source*: adapted from Last, 1995)

Enumeration district (ED)
An area used to disseminate Census data containing roughly 314 people aged under 65. There were 151,000 EDs in Britain in 1991 (those in Scotland are called output areas and there were 38,000 of them). (*Source*: authors)

Life expectancy
The average number of years an individual of a given age is expected to live if current mortality rates continue to apply. (*Source*: adapted from Last, 1995)

Odds ratio
The odds ratio is the ratio of two odds, in this case the odds of disease, death or other outcomes such as living in poverty. It refers to the ratio of the odds of an outcome among those in one group (eg owner-occupiers) to the odds of the outcome among another group (eg those living in social housing). (*Source*: adapted from Last, 1995)

Relative risks
The ratio of the risk of disease or death among those exposed to a particular factor/risk compared to that among the unexposed. (*Source*: adapted from Last, 1995)

Sample of Anonymised Records (SARs)
SARs is a source of individual level data from the 1991 Census that allows tables to be produced which were not originally published. It is derived from two samples: (i) a sample of 2% of all individuals; and (ii) a sample of 1% of households. For each sample far more information was provided than for the SAS (see below). For more details see Dale and Marsh (1993). (*Source*: authors)

Small Area Statistics (SAS)
These are SAS from the 1991 Census (and 1981 Census) available for EDs and larger areas. They include tables of Census statistics either of 100% or 10% of individuals, households or families. For this report 1991 SAS have been aggregated to 1981 wards and 1997 constituencies. For more details see Dale and Marsh (1993). (*Source*: authors)

SMRs – age-sex-Standardised Mortality Ratios
The ratio of the number of deaths observed in the study group or population to the number that would be expected if the study population had the same age-sex-specific rates as the standard population, multiplied by 100. This measure allows groups with different age and sex distributions to be compared. SMRs can also be calculated for the two sexes separately. (*Source*: adapted from Last, 1995)

Social class
The Registrar General's classification of social class is the most commonly used measure of social position in health inequalities research. It classifies people into six classes according to the type of their occupation: I professional; II managerial and technical; IIIN skilled non-manual; IIIM skilled manual; IV partly skilled manual; and V unskilled manual. See Box 2.2 (Chapter 2) for more detail.

Socio-economic group
Socio-economic groups are used to classify people according to their occupation, employment status and also their life-styles in terms of social, cultural and leisure behaviour. It is an aggregate concept based on both resources (material as well as social) and prestige.

Standard population
A population for which the age and sex composition is known. For the data presented here, the standard population is the population of England and Wales, most commonly 1991-95. (*Source*: adapted from Last, 1995)

Ward
A local government ward is an area used to elect councillors, made up of roughly 15 EDs each with an average population of 4,500 people aged under 65. (*Source*: authors)

To Jacob Davey Lambert
born
12 July 1999

Introduction

Inequality in health is the worst inequality of all. There is no more serious inequality than knowing that you'll die sooner because you're badly off. (Frank Dobson/DoH, 1997a)

This book examines and explains a simple fact: that at the end of the 20th century inequalities in health are extremely wide and are still widening in Britain. These inequalities are shown most clearly through the premature deaths of hundreds of thousands of people living in this country over the last two decades. We argue that such inequalities are patently unfair and that inequalities in health are the direct consequence of inequalities in wealth and the growth of poverty in Britain. We also propose that policies to reduce poverty would reduce inequalities in health and that without such fundamental policies we can only expect inequalities in health to continue to widen. However, before we present the evidence of the health gap in Britain, how it has been widening, and, most importantly, what we think should be done about it, it is appropriate to first consider the context of health inequalities and policy in Britain over the past two decades.

From the Black Report to the Independent Inquiry into Inequalities in Health

At the end of the 1970s the previous Labour government appointed Sir Douglas Black to chair a working group to review the evidence on inequalities in health and to suggest policy recommendations that should follow. The report was published (DHSS, 1980) – although with no press release and only 260 copies initially printed. Under the incoming Conservative government in 1980 the Report received a cold reception. A subsequent edition published by Penguin, however, made the findings widely available, and it was later published in conjunction with a later report *The health divide*, which updated the findings (Townsend and Davidson, 1988). The major finding of the Black Report was that there were large differentials in mortality and morbidity that favoured the higher social classes, and that these were not being adequately addressed by health or social services. The Report presented a number of costed policy suggestions, and concluded:

> Above all, we consider that the abolition of child poverty should be adopted as a national goal for the 1980s. (Townsend and Davidson, 1988, p 206)

However, the political will to implement the necessarily redistributive policies that would achieve this goal did not exist at the time. For 17 years in opposition the Labour government made political capital out of the non-implementation of the suggestions of the Black Committee. Before they were elected in May 1997, it was announced that, if elected, Labour would commission an Independent Inquiry into Inequalities in Health, which it duly did in July of 1997, under the chairmanship of Sir Donald Acheson (a former chief medical officer). Tessa Jowell, the Minister for Public Health, criticised the previous administration for "its excessive emphasis on lifestyle issues" which "cast the responsibility back onto the individual" (Jowell/DoH, 1997a). However, despite a commitment that the report of the Inquiry Committee "based on evidence, will contribute to the development of a new strategy for health" (*Independent Inquiry into Inequalities in Health*, 1998) there was also the stipulation that its recommendations should fall within the broad framework of the government's overall financial strategy (see Box 5.1 in Chapter 5). This strategy included maintaining the overall fiscal plans of the previous Conservative administration, at least for the first two years of office.

The report of the Independent Inquiry into Inequalities in Health was published, after some delay, at the end of November 1998. The report contained a comprehensive review of current knowledge on the extent and trends in health inequalities and contained a raft of policy recommendations, many not dissimilar to those in the Black Report. Despite this, however, three key criticisms were levied at the report (Davey Smith et al, 1998a). The first was that there was not adequate prioritisation among the 39 sets of recommendations. Thus the fundamental role of poverty and income differentials was lost in a sea of (albeit worthy) recommendations ranging from traffic curbing to the fluoridation of the water supply.

The second, and related, criticism of the Inquiry's report was that many of the recommendations were simply too vague and decontextualised from the contemporary policy and political agendas to be useful. For example, greater use of and access to public transport was advocated without reference to the price-increasing effects of recent privatisation policies.

The third set of criticisms of the report related more directly to the implementation of the recommendations: the costing of the suggested policies. As the recommendations of the Acheson Report (unlike the Black Report) were not costed, it is impossible to weigh up the costs, benefits and opportunity costs of implementation or inaction. It is thus also impossible to judge the extent to which these suggestions are 'cost-effective' (whatever this was intended to mean), as the remit for the Inquiry requested. (Costings of the recommendations of the Black Report, by the original authors of that report, for both 1982 and 1996 prices, are presented in the Foreword to this book.)

Reducing inequalities in health

Despite its shortcomings, the presence of the Independent Inquiry emphasised the centrality of the issue of health inequalities. The reduction of inequalities in health, and reducing inequalities in general, are core concerns of the Labour government. The government pledged to eliminate childhood poverty by 2019. The Green Paper, *Our healthier nation* (DoH, 1998a) – published before the Inquiry's report – had as one of its aims:

> ... improving the health of the worst off in society and narrowing the health gap.

And the Prime Minister himself pledged:

> I believe in greater equality. If the next Labour Government has not raised the living standards of the poorest by the end of its time in office it will have failed. (Tony Blair, 1996, quoted in Howarth et al, 1998, p 9)

However, the strategy that the Labour government has adopted in order to pursue this goal was somewhat different to that which we might have expected before the 1997 General Election. In *Scotland: The real divide* (1983), on the issue of inequality, Gordon Brown and Robin Cook wrote the following:

This [attaining greater equality] would mean restoring to the centre of the tax system two basic principals: the first, that those who cannot afford to pay tax should not have to pay it; and the second, that taxation should rise progressively with income. Programmes that merely redistribute poverty from families to single persons, from the old to the young, from the sick to the healthy, are not a solution. What is needed, is a programme of reform that ends the current situation where the top 10% own 80% of our wealth and 30% of income, even after tax. As Tawney remarked, 'What some people call the problem of poverty, others call the problem of riches'. (Brown and Cook, 1983, p 22)

A statement by government Minister Stephen Byers showed how the Labour Party has moved away from this notion of redistribution through direct taxation over the last 16 years:

The reality is that wealth creation is now more important than wealth redistribution. (Stephen Byers, Minister for Trade and Industry, quoted in Jones, 1999)

New Labour believed that the income raised from economic growth could be used to eradicate poverty, and that redistribution as we have known it in the past – through increasing the tax burden of the better-off and raising benefits and incomes in real terms for the poorer – should no longer be seen as the key policy option.

Instead, policies focused on getting people into work or increasing the incomes of those already in work (eg Welfare to Work, the Minimum Wage, Working Families Tax Credit) were welcomed. However, as we show in this book, the majority of those living on very low incomes are not in work and could not take work even if more work were available (because they are caring for children and other dependants or are over retirement age). Policies which target only a small proportion of the population (eg Health Action Zones, Employment Action Zones, Sure Start) will only reach a small proportion of those in need. In addition, bringing pensions and benefit changes in line with changes in average earnings does not reduce inequalities, it simply maintains them. It is therefore our concern that the Labour government elected in 1997, while laudable in its aims, will not have a substantial effect on inequalities in Britain.

The widening gap

This book is driven by our concern about the increasing inequality of health outcomes. In the following four chapters we present our own review of the current extent of health inequalities in Britain and what should be done about them.

Chapter 2 presents new evidence of the extent of the health gap. The Black Report and its successor contained a vast array of evidence, but we update this further. For example, whereas the report of the Independent Inquiry referred to mortality by social class for the years 1991-93, we include data referring to the period 1992-96. These data show that the social class mortality gap is even wider than previously thought. For instance, the life expectancy gap between men in social class I (professional occupations) and social class V (unskilled manual occupations) is now a staggering 9.5 years; for women it is 6.4 years (Hattersley, 1999). The health gap between different communities also widened as the Acheson Committee was sitting (the Inquiry did not address geographical inequalities).

We also have a broader scope, in that we include a geographical dimension in our analysis. We present the first geographical data on mortality at the constituency level for the whole of Britain. We compare the fortunes of people living in the constituencies containing the one million people with the highest mortality rates, with the fortunes of the one million people in constituencies with the lowest mortality rates. The difference is such that death rates for the 'worst health' million are 2.6 times those for the 'best health' million. Had the mortality ratios of the 'worst health' million been the same as the 'best health' million then 71% of the deaths under 65 would not have occurred in the period 1991-95. We compare these 'best health' and 'worst health' constituencies as we consider the health gap and the socio-economic gap which underlies it through different stages of the life-course. We show how in contemporary Britain unequal chances of death are interwoven, in social and spatial terms, with unequal chances in life, in terms of education, employment, income and wealth.

In Chapter 3 we move beyond description of the health gap and review explanations for the health gap and the evidence for these. We show how recent research has demonstrated that social circumstances across the entire life-course – from birth through to late adulthood – influence people's health and well-being. In addition, the characteristics of the areas in which people live, as well as their individual characteristics, are shown to be important in influencing their health. While factors such as education and behaviours such as smoking are important factors in producing health inequalities, we show that health differentials are primarily related to the long-term material well-being of social groups, not to the psychosocial effects of position in hierarchies. Reduction of inequalities in health cannot be brought about by people feeling better about their (unfair) lot in the world – only the redistribution of material resources will produce such a reduction.

In Chapter 4, we present evidence of the extent to which the social and spatial health gap in Britain has widened over the past two decades, and that this polarisation has mirrored socio-economic widening, primarily in the form of increased income inequality and increased poverty. Britain has experienced some of the fastest growth in income inequality in the developed world and by the late 1990s had some of the highest levels of poverty seen within Europe. We also demonstrate that widening inequality is not inevitable and that these differentials narrowed in the 1960s and 1970s. Just as the gap can widen, so it can narrow. This chapter illustrates the possible consequences of inadequate policies. The trends of growing inequality show no signs of abating and the consequences of such a widening gap are dire.

In the final chapter we present the policy options that we consider to be essential if inequalities in health are to be tackled. We also address the convoluted policy debate on inequalities in health. Here we have a simple message: the key policy that will reduce inequalities in health is the alleviation of poverty through the reduction in income and wealth inequality. We show how there is widespread public support for poverty reduction in Britain. We argue that poverty can be reduced by raising the standards of living of poor people through increasing their incomes 'in cash' or 'in kind'. The costs would be borne by the rich and would reduce inequalities overall – simultaneously reducing inequalities in health. It is our firm belief that if the health inequalities which are described and explained in this book are to be reduced, as is the stated aim of the government, then policies which actively and actually address the reduction of poverty and the reduction of inequality through redistribution must be pursued.

In short the structure of this book has been made as simple as possible. We produce evidence that the extent of the health gap is wider than official reports suggest (Chapter 2). We present the most up-to-date evidence of the causes of those inequalities in health (Chapter 3). We provide clear statistical evidence as to how the health gap is continuing to widen, but how it has not always done so (Chapter 4). And we have prepared and argued for an alternative policy agenda (Chapter 5), which, if you accept the overall picture presented in earlier chapters, would narrow the health gap.

TWO

The health gap

Summary

This chapter provides evidence of the geographical and social inequalities in health in contemporary Britain. We compare the extreme areas of Britain – using parliamentary constituencies as the geographical unit – with the lowest and highest premature mortality. We compare life chances in these areas through stages of the life-course:

- Infant mortality is 2.0 times more likely in the 'worst health' compared to the 'best health' constituencies.

- In the 'worst health' constituencies 4.2 times as many households with children live in poverty compared to the 'best health' constituencies.

- In the 'worst health' constituencies GCSE failure rates are 1.5 times higher and post-school qualifications are half the rate of those in the 'best health' constituencies.

- There are more people in social classes IV and V and less in social classes I and II in the 'worst health' constituencies than the 'best health' constituencies but this only partially accounts for the health differences between those areas.

- The 'worst health' constituencies have 3.6 times as many people not working and 2.8 times as many people with a limiting long-term illness as compared to the 'best health' constituencies.

- Average household incomes in the 'worst health' constituencies are 70% of those in the 'best health' constituencies.

- The 'best health' constituencies have 9.1 times more households with 3 or more cars and 6.5 times more households with 7 or more rooms than the 'worst health' constituencies.

- In the 'worst health' constituencies women aged 75-84 are 60% less likely to be married than those in the 'best health' constituencies because men there are more likely to die relatively early in life.

Introduction

This chapter presents evidence of the health gap in Britain and how health varies between different social groups in different areas. It shows these inequalities by travelling through the life-course, highlighting the social, political and economic factors that influence people's health as they age. We show that mortality and illness (morbidity) are highest in localities which also have high rates of poverty, unemployment and other manifestations of social and economic deprivation.

In this chapter we refer to some sources of secondary data but our main source of evidence is new data for geographical areas in Britain. Much of the readily available information on health inequalities applies only to England and Wales. This is because official statistics treat Scotland differently and because the Office for National Statistics (ONS) Longitudinal Study (LS), one of the main sources of data on this topic, does not include Scotland. This omission can make the health gap appear to be more narrow than it really is. Fortunately, geographical data on morbidity and mortality are available for all parts of Britain and so we use these to describe geographical variations in life chances. We will use rates in England and Wales to standardise these statistics so that our new figures are comparable with official publications. However, as almost no information is readily available on Northern Ireland, disaggregated by area or class, we have omitted that area.

The geography of mortality

The new data presented refer to parliamentary constituencies and have been calculated from individual mortality records. We have chosen to use parliamentary constituencies to illustrate the extent of the health gap in Britain because constituencies are of roughly equal population size, are readily identifiable, are represented by democratically elected politicians who should have their constituents' interests at heart and are, from 1997, relatively stable geographical units. Finally, constituencies are also small enough to encapsulate localities with similar socio-economic experiences: people's lives are shaped by the places they currently live in as well as by the places they have lived in in the past. For instance, in some parts of Britain finding work is still relatively unproblematic, while in other places unemployment is common. In some areas the majority of children will go to university because of the schools in those areas and because the wealth and expectations of their parents, friends and neighbours enables and encourages them to do this.

These children are those most likely to enter the professions and reap the health benefits that accompany affluence. In time, they tend to settle and raise families in the same kinds of areas as their parents did and this helps to maintain and strengthen a cycle of privilege that is manifest through the places where people live.

Poorer children, on the other hand, will usually be born to families living in areas where almost no children from local schools will go to university, where there are consequently lower expectations and almost never the wealth which tends to ease people's passage through life, beginning with the benefit of wealth for aiding educational attainment. For young people in poorer areas, the chances of gaining skilled employment are very much lower than for the children of the affluent. Without skilled employment or inherited wealth, their chances of leaving areas like this are constrained by the housing market. In time, this new generation is likely to have their own children within the town and even estate in which they were born and thus maintain this cycle of wealth (and poverty).

The extremes of Britain

To illustrate the size of the health gap between constituencies and the other socio-economic gaps which cause and are a consequence of poor health, the one million people living in constituencies with the 'best health' will be compared with the one million people living in constituencies with the 'worst health'. This is an arbitrary divide but each group contains enough people to ensure that the statistics shown are not the product of random events. The population aged under 65 has been used because it is for this group that the greatest scope to narrow the health gap exists. The most robust and most direct measure of the health gap is premature mortality and so those areas with the highest and lowest premature mortality ratios will be referred to consistently from here on, illustrating the current size of the geographical gap and its growth. For brevity we will also refer to the people living within these constituencies as those with the 'best health' and 'worst health'.

If the million people with the 'best health' were compared with the million people with the 'worst health', according to the local government ward they lived in, the gap would be found to be very large indeed. However, wards are often too small to encompass whole communities and there would not be sufficient space to list all the hundreds of wards involved. Instead, 1997 parliamentary constituencies have been used here to illustrate the extent of the current health gap in Britain. Parliamentary constituencies are of roughly equal population sizes (containing an average of 74,000 people under the age of 65) and are small enough to group into areas of one million people. Mortality over the period 1991 to 1995 is considered, using the latest data available, which are also comparable to past data for the period 1981-85 – from when the gap began to widen most (data on the widening gap are presented in Chapter 4). Box 2.1 provides a summary of this method.

Box 2.1: Comparing the extreme health areas of Britain

Source of data:	Office for National Statistics (ONS) and General Register Office (Scotland) digital mortality records
Geographical units:	Constituencies, using 1997 boundaries
Population included:	All those under 65 using mid-year estimates
Years covered:	1991-95 to show the extent of the current gap, comparing 1981-95 to 1991-95 to show the widening gap
Health measure:	SMRs for deaths under 65
'Worst health' million:	The 15 constituencies, with the population under 65 totalling approximately one million, with the highest SMRs
'Best health' million:	The 13 constituencies, with the population under 65 totalling approximately one million, with the lowest SMRs
Other sources of data:	The Population Censuses of Britain carried out in 1981 and 1991. The *Breadline Britain* survey of 1,831 adults carried out in 1990. School exam performance data from the Department of Education and Employment (DfEE), and the Welsh and Scottish Offices

Note: Appendix A presents the ranked SMRs under 65 for all 641 of the 1997 constituencies.

Table 2.1 lists the 15 parliamentary constituencies which contain the million people aged under 65 with the highest and lowest age-sex-standardised mortality ratios (SMRs) in Britain between 1991 and 1995 (see Glossary). The highest ratio was in Glasgow Shettleston, where the chances of dying at any time under age 65 are 2.3 times the national average. Had the mortality ratios of this constituency been the same as for those of the 'best health' one million people, 71% of the deaths of constituents under 65 would not have occurred in the period under study. Overall, for the areas containing the million people with the 'worst health', 10,921 would still be alive if they enjoyed the mortality rates of the million people with the 'best health' over just five years – this represents nearly two thirds of all deaths under 65 in these constituencies. The second half of the table shows the very low mortality rates that are enjoyed by people living in the 'best health' areas that together contain one million people. As we go on to show throughout this book, it is the conditions in which people can afford to live, given current market and political arrangements, which determine who lives to an old age and who dies young.

Figure 2.1 presents data on the extent of the geographical gap in map form. The clustering of the 'worst health' areas of Britain in Glasgow, the northern conurbations and in the centre of London is made starkly clear. Even among these 'worst health' one million people, a north to south gradient in mortality ratios is apparent. In all these areas mortality ratios are very high, but they range from 2.3 times average at their worst in Glasgow, to 1.6 times average in Southwark and Bermondsey. Conversely, there is much less variation between the million people with the 'best health' in Britain. The position of constituencies across the south of England shows remarkable uniformity of rates suggesting that there are no particularly 'special' factors causing mortality rates to be so low in these areas – other than general affluence. The pattern is broken by Sheffield Hallam constituency – illustrating how low mortality ratios in the north could be.

Table 2.1: **Constituencies where people are most and least at risk of premature death (mortality rates under 65) in Britain (1991-95)**

Rank	Name	Obs<65	SMR<65	Pop<65	Avoidable
Ratio of 'worst health' to 'best health'		2.3	2.6	1.0	
1	Glasgow Shettleston	1,405	234	50,740	71%
2	Glasgow Springburn	1,438	217	57,007	69%
3	Glasgow Maryhill	1,432	196	67,246	65%
4	Glasgow Pollok	1,313	187	62,257	64%
5	Glasgow Anniesland	1,176	181	56,757	63%
6	Glasgow Baillieston	1,267	180	66,076	62%
7	Manchester Central	1,597	173	94,191	61%
8	Glasgow Govan	1,028	172	57,286	61%
9	Liverpool Riverside	1,458	172	83,267	61%
10	Manchester Blackley	1,421	169	78,573	60%
11	Greenock and Inverclyde	1,051	164	54,050	59%
12	Salford	1,285	163	72,681	59%
13	Tyne Bridge	1,297	158	76,678	57%
14	Glasgow Kelvin	828	158	50,304	57%
15	Southwark North and Bermondsey	1,214	156	76,811	56%
'Worst health' million		*19,210*	*178*	*1,003,923*	*62%*

Rank	Name	Obs<65	SMR<65	Pop<65
1	Wokingham	588	65	80,936
2	Woodspring	620	65	74,251
3	Romsey	593	65	73,300
4	Sheffield Hallam	481	66	61,865
5	South Cambridgeshire	636	66	79,401
6	Chesham and Amersham	673	67	76,914
7	South Norfolk	710	69	79,820
8	West Chelmsford	674	69	83,988
9	South Suffolk	601	69	68,686
10	Witney	675	69	82,975
11	Esher and Walton	705	69	83,333
12	Northavon	742	70	88,333
13	Buckingham	593	71	70,344
'Best health' million		*8,291*	*68*	*1,004,147*
Britain		**556,957**	**100**	**47,587,310**

Notes: The population of each constituency is estimated for 1993 from 1991 mid-year ward statistics updated by the 1996 ONS age/sex mid-year estimates of population for local authority districts. The mortality figures are assigned to constituencies through the postcodes of the deceased.

Source: Analysis by authors

Obs<65	Number of deaths under the age of 65
SMR<65	Standardised Mortality Ratio for deaths under 65
Pop<65	Number of people in the constituency under the age of 65
Avoidable	% of deaths which would not have occurred if the 'worst health' areas had the death rate of the 'best health' areas

Figure 2.1: **Premature deaths in the extreme areas of Britain (1991-95)**

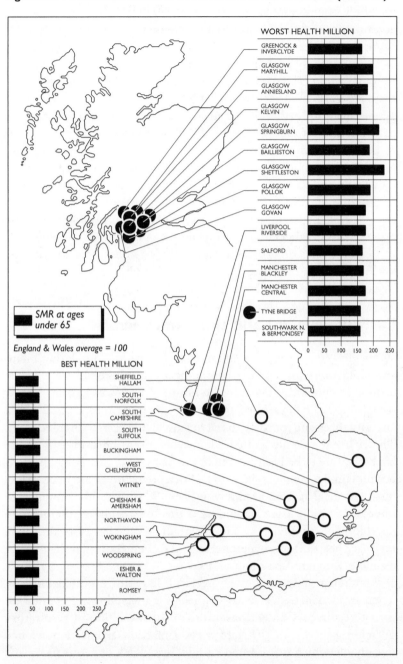

Source: Table 2.1

The geography of the areas with the highest and lowest mortality ratios under 65 requires more comment. Just over half of these 'worst health' constituencies are in Glasgow (and one more is also on the Clyde). Scottish and urban constituencies tend to be smaller than average but, even if we were to take this into account, it would have little impact on the distribution. This is because many of the constituencies neighbouring these areas also have very poor health and 52% of the worst off million people in terms of health live in Scotland. Of the remainder of the constituencies of the 'worst health' million, three are contiguous areas in central Manchester, containing 24% of the 'worst health' million people in Britain. The other three areas – in the centres of Liverpool, Newcastle and London – contain an equal proportion of the 'worst health' million (24%). These are the inner areas of some of Britain's largest cities. Expanding the list to over one million would bring in the poorest parts of other cities (see Appendix A which lists all constituencies in million group order). By contrast, the 13 constituencies with the lowest mortality ratios are all, save Sheffield Hallam, in the south of Britain and mainly in suburban and rural areas.

Early life – infant and child mortality

We begin our journey through the life-course by considering infant and child mortality. At the beginning of life there are clear socio-economic differences between the health of babies in Britain. This is true both for babies born to families in poorer individual social circumstances, and for babies born to families living in poorer localities. The richer the family and community a child is born into, the more likely they are to be healthy, even in the first year of life. Babies born to poorer families are more likely to be born prematurely and to be of low birth weight (MacFarlane and Mugford, 1984). This has a number of important implications, including a greater likelihood of impaired development, cerebral palsy, and of certain chronic diseases – including coronary heart disease, hypertension and diabetes – in later life (see, for example, Kuh and Ben-Shlomo, 1997).

Children in poorer families are more likely to experience illness. There is evidence of a social gradient for the following conditions: infant respiratory infections/bronchiolitis, childhood respiratory infection, gastroenteritis, *Helicobacter pylori* infection (an infection acquired in early life which is associated with increased risk of peptic ulcers and stomach cancer in later life), dental caries, tuberculosis and HIV (Reading, 1997a). A study of *Helicobacter pylori* infection in children, for example, found that it was more likely to be found in children from overcrowded homes, in single-parent families, in rented rather than owned homes and in children attending schools which were classed as having a deprived catchment area (Patel et al, 1994). There is also a clear social class gradient for limiting long-term illness (LLTI), as measured in the Census (Gordon and Heslop, 1999), such that there are 1.4 times as many children with a LLTI in social class V families as would be expected had they had the average rate of illness for all children. In terms of mortality, injury and poisoning is now the major category of cause of death for children. Although the overall rates of death from these causes have been falling in the past couple of decades, children whose parents do unskilled manual work are now five times more likely to die from injury or poisoning than are children whose parents have professional occupations (Roberts and Power, 1996).

Table 2.2 refers to the same 'best health' and 'worst health' constituencies referred to above, but shows the infant and child mortality rates for these areas. The table shows that infant mortality rates are 2.0 times higher for those in the highest mortality constituencies compared to the lowest mortality constituencies, 2.0 times higher for deaths to children aged 1 to 4 and 1.8 times higher for children aged 5 to 14. The final two columns of the table give the total number of children aged under 15 who died in these constituencies over the five years 1991-95 and the total number of children at risk. Although the numbers dying are small, nationally some 34,000 children died over this period, over 1,000 of these children died in the 'worst health' areas, compared to less than 500 in the 'best health' areas – despite the overall numbers of children at risk being nearly identical. Figure 2.2 shows the infant mortality rates from this table on the map of Britain. Each coffin represents one baby in a thousand dying in the first year of life. At the most extreme, for every baby that died in Woodspring, four died in Southwark North and Bermondsey.

The risks faced by our children are thus clearly strongly linked to their social and spatial circumstances. As Reading has said:

> The links between poverty and child health are extensive, strong, and pervasive ... virtually all aspects of health are worst among children living in poverty than among children from affluent families. (Reading, 1997b, p 463)

Table 2.2: **Infant and child mortality rates per 10,000 per year by age in the extreme areas of Britain (1991-95)**

Rank	Name	Rate aged 0	Rate aged 1 to 4	Rate aged 5 to 14	Obs 0-14	Pop 0-14
Ratio of 'worst health' to 'best health' areas		**2.0**	**2.0**	**1.8**	**2.2**	**1.0**
1	Glasgow Shettleston	109.7	3.9	1.5	57	10,443
2	Glasgow Springburn	67.9	3.4	2.8	49	12,156
3	Glasgow Maryhill	72.6	4.1	2.2	55	13,988
4	Glasgow Pollok	84.9	2.3	2.2	57	15,081
5	Glasgow Anniesland	103.0	4.0	2.2	61	12,533
6	Glasgow Baillieston	80.4	6.3	3.1	77	16,762
7	Manchester Central	88.6	5.5	1.8	111	23,383
8	Glasgow Govan	86.1	7.2	2.1	62	11,813
9	Liverpool Riverside	62.9	4.0	2.9	68	17,859
10	Manchester Blackley	69.9	4.7	2.2	84	20,957
11	Greenock and Inverclyde	94.1	4.1	0.5	44	12,213
12	Salford	73.0	7.2	2.4	78	17,023
13	Tyne Bridge	106.3	3.1	1.4	89	18,013
14	Glasgow Kelvin	54.9	2.2	2.0	20	6,392
15	Southwark North and Bermondsey	124.6	5.6	1.8	121	17,291
'Worst health' million		*86.4*	*4.7*	*2.1*	*1,033*	*225,907*
Rank	**Name**					
1	Wokingham	53.2	2.0	1.2	46	18,363
2	Woodspring	30.0	2.0	0.9	23	16,321
3	Romsey	54.3	0.5	1.1	33	16,253
4	Sheffield Hallam	39.1	3.9	2.0	28	11,979
5	South Cambridgeshire	41.1	2.7	2.0	40	17,241
6	Chesham and Amersham	38.2	2.9	1.0	33	17,070
7	South Norfolk	35.7	2.8	1.4	33	16,902
8	West Chelmsford	42.0	1.6	0.5	36	18,445
9	South Suffolk	46.0	1.6	1.1	30	15,354
10	Witney	39.4	3.4	1.3	44	18,530
11	Esher and Walton	51.6	1.9	0.5	41	18,851
12	Northavon	47.9	2.6	1.4	49	19,700
13	Buckingham	38.0	2.9	1.1	32	16,175
'Best health' million		*43.2*	*2.3*	*1.2*	*468*	*221,184*
Britain		63.3	3.1	1.6	34,025	10,767,181

Source: Analysis by authors

Rate aged 0	Death rate per 10,000 in first year of life
Rate aged 1 to 4	Death rate per 10,000 for ages 1 to 4 inclusive
Rate aged 5 to 14	Death rate per 10,000 for ages 5 to 14 inclusive
Obs 0-14	Total number of deaths of children aged 0 to 14 inclusive
Pop 0-14	Total number of children aged 0 to 14 inclusive

Figure 2.2: **Infant mortality rates in the extreme areas of Britain (1991-95)**

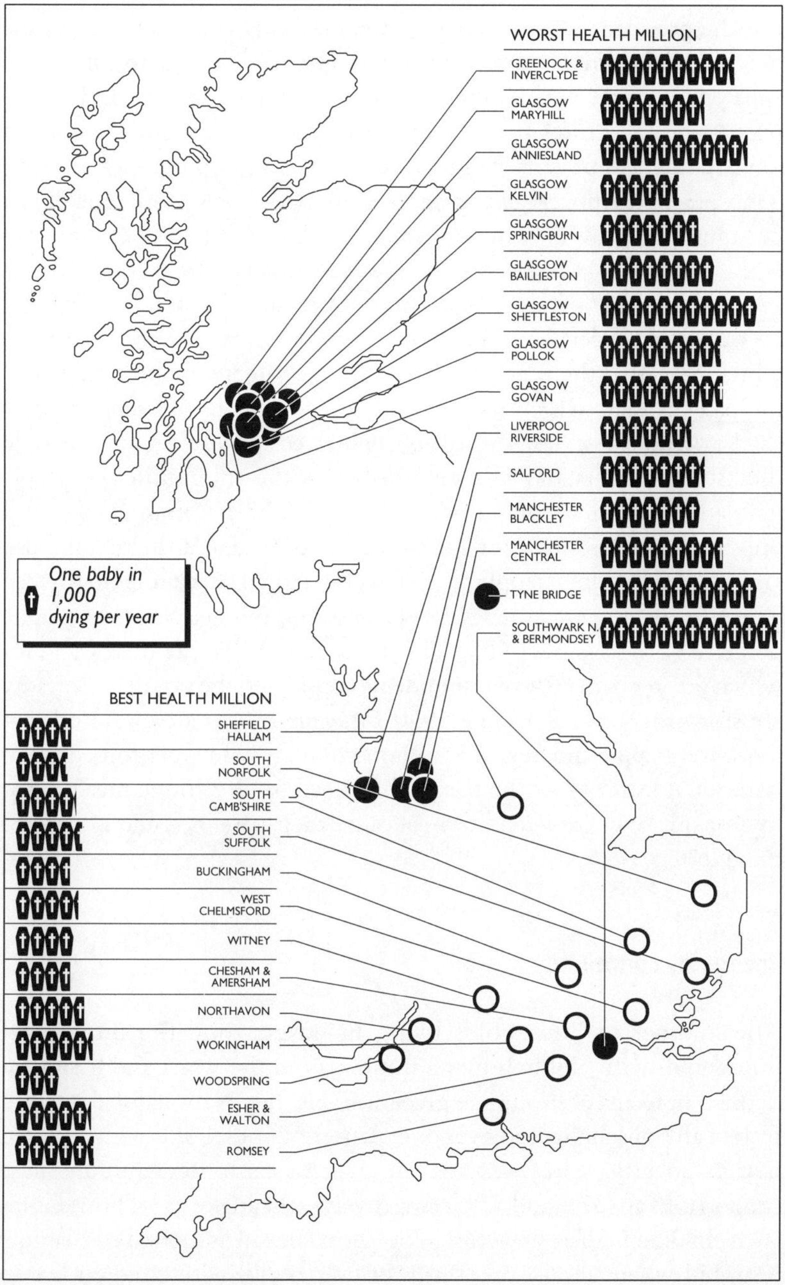

WORST HEALTH MILLION

GREENOCK & INVERCLYDE	
GLASGOW MARYHILL	
GLASGOW ANNIESLAND	
GLASGOW KELVIN	
GLASGOW SPRINGBURN	
GLASGOW BAILLIESTON	
GLASGOW SHETTLESTON	
GLASGOW POLLOK	
GLASGOW GOVAN	
LIVERPOOL RIVERSIDE	
SALFORD	
MANCHESTER BLACKLEY	
MANCHESTER CENTRAL	
TYNE BRIDGE	
SOUTHWARK N. & BERMONDSEY	

One baby in 1,000 dying per year

BEST HEALTH MILLION

SHEFFIELD HALLAM	
SOUTH NORFOLK	
SOUTH CAMB'SHIRE	
SOUTH SUFFOLK	
BUCKINGHAM	
WEST CHELMSFORD	
WITNEY	
CHESHAM & AMERSHAM	
NORTHAVON	
WOKINGHAM	
WOODSPRING	
ESHER & WALTON	
ROMSEY	

Source: Table 2.2

Childhood poverty

It is the prevalence of poverty in childhood in Britain that leads to the differential health outcomes of babies and young children being so apparent. Poverty means different things to different people and debate over what constitutes poverty and how it can be measured has been long-standing as poverty has developed from an 'absolute' to a 'relative' concept. While poverty has been measured by levels of income, it can be argued that poverty can only accurately be described by referring to living standards. Here we use the *Breadline Britain* survey conducted in 1990 as a measure of poverty (see Appendix B and Gordon and Pantazis, 1997, for more details). The *Breadline Britain* surveys and the surveys which preceded them are the only nationally representative studies in the past 25 years which have considered poverty in this sense as they used a measure of 'consensual' or 'perceived' poverty – what people themselves understand and experience as the minimum acceptable standard of living in contemporary Britain. This minimum covers not only the basic essentials for survival, such as food and shelter, but also factors which enable people to participate in their social roles in society. The survey thus measured what possessions and activities the public perceived as necessities of life. The items included in the survey and for which greater than 50% of respondents considered the item as a necessity are shown in Table 2.3. The 1990 *Breadline Britain* survey found that there were approximately 2.5 million children who were forced to go without at least one of the things they need (such as three meals a day, toys or out-of-school activities), because their parents could not afford these things.

Poverty by community

The number of households living in poverty and the number of households with children living in poverty in the worst and best areas defined in terms of health are given in Table 2.4. Nationally just over a fifth of all households and over one quarter of households with children live in poverty. However, for the 'worst health' one million these proportions are 37% and 53% respectively – the majority of households with children in these areas live in poverty. The rate is highest in Glasgow Maryhill where almost two thirds of households with children live in poverty. For the 'best health' one million people only 13% of households in their areas live in poverty and the proportion is slightly smaller for households with children. Households with children are four times more likely to be living in poverty in the 'worst health' areas as compared to the 'best health' areas. Given this, the wide variation in infant and childhood health is hardly surprising. If anything it is surprising that the differences found are not wider. The table is illustrated in Figure 2.3 which both emphasises just how different the lives of people living in these two groups of areas are and shows that there are still variations between these individual areas.

Table 2.3: **The perception of necessities and % of population having each item: the 1990** *Breadline Britain* **survey**

Standard-of-living items in rank order	% claiming item as necessity (1,831)	% of population having item
A damp-free home	98	94
Heating to warm living areas of the home if it's cold	97	96
An inside toilet (not shared with another household)	97	98
Bath, not shared with another household	95	97
Beds for everyone in the household	95	97
A decent state of decoration in the home	92	81
Fridge	92	98
Warm waterproof coat	91	91
Three meals a day (for children)	90	74
Two meals a day (for adults)	90	94
Insurance of contents of dwelling	88	83
Daily fresh fruit and vegetables	88	88
Toys for children eg dolls or models	84	75
Bedrooms for every child over 10 of different sexes	82	65
Carpets in living rooms and bedrooms	78	96
Meat/fish (or vegetarian equivalent) every other day	77	90
Two pairs all-weather shoes	74	90
Celebrations on special occasions	74	91
Washing machine	73	88
Presents for friends or family once a year	69	90
Child's participation in out-of-school activities	69	50
Regular savings of £10 a month for 'rainy days' or retirement	68	60
Hobby or leisure activity	67	76
New, not second-hand, clothes	65	84
Weekly roast/vegetarian equivalent	64	84
Leisure equipment for children eg sports equipment or bicycle	61	67
A television	58	97
A telephone	56	87
An annual week's holiday away, not with relatives	54	65
A 'best outfit' for special occasions	54	85
An outing for children once a week	53	58
Children's friends round for tea/snack fortnightly	52	55

Source: Gordon and Pantazis (1997)

What Table 2.4 does not account for are the services that are provided by central and local government to reduce the impact of poverty on children. Although infants are four times more likely to be living in poverty in the 'worst health' areas, they are 'only' twice as likely to die before their first birthday. A National Health Service, free at the point of delivery, helps to reduce the effects of poverty on child health. The universal provision of midwives and health visitors and free prescriptions for children all help to reduce the effects of childhood poverty, but do not eliminate them. Most importantly, the magnitude of the health gap for children is only half of that of the poverty gap, by area, because government policies reduce the impact of poverty on children to a great extent. Universal child allowances and no tax on children's clothing are just two examples of state benefits and exceptions which do more to aid the poor than the rich. Free school meals and family credit are other examples. Some of the actions of government help to reduce inequalities in health, but they are not enough to eliminate those inequalities.

Education – inequalities between children

An important stage in the life-course, not least because it is a channel to advantages in later life, is education. The number of children who attended state schools in each of the selected constituencies between 1993 and 1996 and their chance of *not* achieving 5 GCSE exams grade A to C each year are shown in Table 2.5. These can be seen as a current benchmark for assessing educational attainment as these are the basic qualifications needed to enter most skilled jobs later in life. Although the rates in the 'worst health' constituencies improved each year, in line with the national improvement, by 1996 two thirds of the children in these areas were still failing to achieve this level of qualification compared to only 44% failing in state schools in the 'best health' constituencies. In Salford over 80% of children who attend state schools in that constituency fail at this basic level of examination. The education gap is not as wide as the health gap, but there are a number of factors which influence this. Firstly, had we taken a more narrow definition of failure, say, children who fail to gain any GCSEs, then the gap would be wider. Secondly, not all children are included in these statistics. In the richer areas many more children attend private schools where failure rates tend to be very low, whereas in the poorer areas the numbers of expulsions from school are rising and hence more children do not complete their education. Thirdly, and for the same reasons given for the benefits of broader government interventions outlined above, we would not expect the gap in the state-provided service to be as wide as that for health outcomes. Differences in health are much more than the product of inequalities in the provision of state services – they are largely the product of the unequal distribution of income and wealth. The map which illustrates these statistics (Figure 2.4) reinforces how inequalities in education are much narrower than in health.

Table 2.4: **Poverty rates for constituencies where people are most at risk of premature death in Britain (1991)**

Rank	Name	Households	% in poverty	Number in poverty	% with children in poverty	Number with children in poverty
	Ratio of 'worst health' to 'best health'	**1.1**	**2.8**	**3.0**	**4.2**	**3.8**
1	Glasgow Shettleston	25,822	42	10,871	59	3,739
2	Glasgow Springburn	29,646	41	12,244	60	4,522
3	Glasgow Maryhill	28,829	41	11,964	63	4,657
4	Glasgow Pollok	26,238	36	9,498	52	4,191
5	Glasgow Anniesland	27,465	34	9,448	51	3,545
6	Glasgow Baillieston	26,866	39	10,424	54	5,237
7	Manchester Central	38,032	40	15,213	59	6,703
8	Glasgow Govan	27,777	31	8,722	46	3,038
9	Liverpool Riverside	38,038	39	14,873	57	5,747
10	Manchester Blackley	36,199	34	12,199	49	5,596
11	Greenock and Inverclyde	25,490	31	7,902	43	3,332
12	Salford	34,249	34	11,713	48	4,422
13	Tyne Bridge	37,202	37	13,839	55	5,775
14	Glasgow Kelvin	27,741	30	8,239	38	1,664
15	Southwark North and Bermondsey	39,386	38	15,006	57	5,660
	'Worst health' million	*468,980*	*37*	*172,155*	*53*	*67,828*
Rank	**Name**					
1	Wokingham	31,794	10	3,084	9	1,070
2	Woodspring	33,617	11	3,866	12	1,222
3	Romsey	31,702	12	3,931	12	1,264
4	Sheffield Hallam	28,782	15	4,231	9	701
5	South Cambridgeshire	33,590	14	4,837	13	1,374
6	Chesham and Amersham	33,237	11	3,789	11	1,162
7	South Norfolk	37,612	14	5,228	15	1,551
8	West Chelmsford	37,568	15	5,485	16	1,881
9	South Suffolk	32,669	15	4,933	17	1,718
10	Witney	35,412	15	5,241	17	1,886
11	Esher and Walton	38,063	13	4,796	12	1,370
12	Northavon	36,083	11	3,933	11	1,368
13	Buckingham	29,276	13	3,718	11	1,135
	'Best health' million	*439,405*	*13*	*57,072*	*13*	*17,702*
Britain		21,619,998	21	4,501,356	27	1,744,872

Source: Analysis by authors, from the *Breadline Britain* survey and 1991 Census

Figure 2.3: **Poverty rates of households with children in the extreme areas of Britain (1991)**

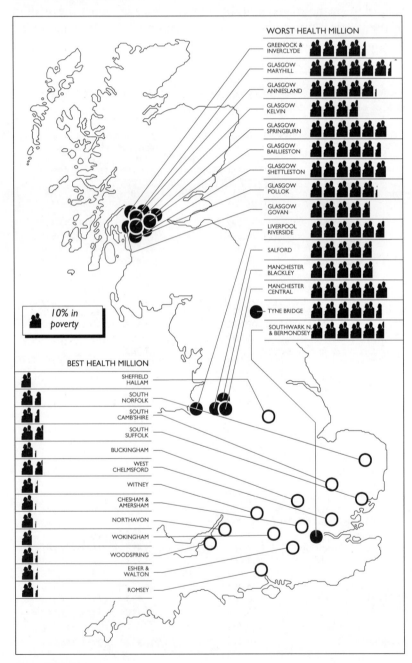

Source: Table 2.4

Moving on to what for many young people today is the next stage in the life-course, Table 2.6 shows the proportions of adults who reported having post-school qualifications in the 1991 Census. Because, until recently, we educated only a small proportion of people beyond school level, these statistics are shown per thousand rather than as percentages. In Britain as a whole less than one in a hundred (0.9%) of adults have a higher degree; 6.2% have a degree and 6.3% have a diploma. Of all adults with at least one of these qualifications only 0.4% were unemployed or on a government scheme in 1991. Education is clearly one of the best means of avoiding unemployment and poverty, although access to post-school education is largely determined by social class rather than ability. Because of this social entry selection and later migration, more than twice as many adults living in the 'best health' areas of Britain have these qualifications compared to those in the 'worst health' areas in Britain. Furthermore, adults in the 'worst health' areas are 49% more likely to be unemployed even if they have these qualifications than those in the 'best health' areas, but the unemployment rate of this group in the 'worst health' areas is still only 0.6%.

When we map the absolute numbers of people who have university degrees (multiplying the second and last columns of Table 2.6 and dividing by 1,000), part of the reason for inequalities in higher education being relatively low becomes clear (see Figure 2.5). A few of the 'worst health' constituencies are located near major universities and that leads to high variations within the 'worst health' group. Ten times as many people have degrees in Glasgow Kelvin as in Glasgow Baillieston, for example.

Table 2.5: **GCSE failure* rates for constituencies where people are most and least at risk of premature death in Britain (1993-96)**

Rank	Name	Pupils 1993-96	% in 1993	% in 1994	% in 1995	% in 1996
	Ratio of 'worst health' to 'best health' areas		1.5	1.6	1.5	1.5
1	Glasgow Shettleston	3,361	62	65	61	57
2	Glasgow Springburn	2,554	82	78	79	77
3	Glasgow Maryhill	1,908	77	77	72	70
4	Glasgow Pollok	2,569	70	68	65	67
5	Glasgow Anniesland	2,222	64	60	60	60
6	Glasgow Baillieston	2,733	72	69	65	65
7	Manchester Central	1,701	79	72	73	69
8	Glasgow Govan	2,298	70	65	65	69
9	Liverpool Riverside	3,160	70	72	69	70
10	Manchester Blackley	4,594	82	80	77	74
11	Greenock and Inverclyde	3,319	53	51	49	49
12	Salford	2,912	82	84	80	81
13	Tyne Bridge	2,314	65	66	57	52
14	Glasgow Kelvin	2,761	62	60	59	57
15	Southwark North and Bermondsey	3,343	83	83	75	70
	'Worst health' million	*41,749*	*72*	*70*	*67*	*66*
Rank	**Name**					
1	Wokingham	5,393	48	43	45	46
2	Woodspring	3,902	48	41	41	39
3	Romsey	5,445	49	44	43	44
4	Sheffield Hallam	5,096	49	44	45	42
5	South Cambridgeshire	3,976	49	42	41	40
6	Chesham and Amersham	4,828	40	38	41	41
7	South Norfolk	4,457	50	48	44	46
8	West Chelmsford	4,831	42	41	37	38
9	South Suffolk	3,373	50	48	46	45
10	Witney	4,056	52	50	50	50
11	Esher and Walton	1,694	60	57	58	62
12	Northavon	4,193	52	47	48	49
13	Buckingham	2,102	58	53	47	48
	'Best health' million	*53,346*	*49*	*45*	*44*	*44*
Britain		2,355,272	61	59	58	57

Note: in Scotland Scottish Ordinary level exam grades 1 to 3 are assumed equivalent to GCSE grade A to C. * 'Failure' is defined as not achieving 5 GCSE exams grade A to C. Pupils 1993-96 are numbers of pupils taking these exams over this period, % are those failing each year.

Source: Analysis by authors from school exam results tables

Figure 2.4: **GCSE failure rates in the extreme areas of Britain (1991-95)**

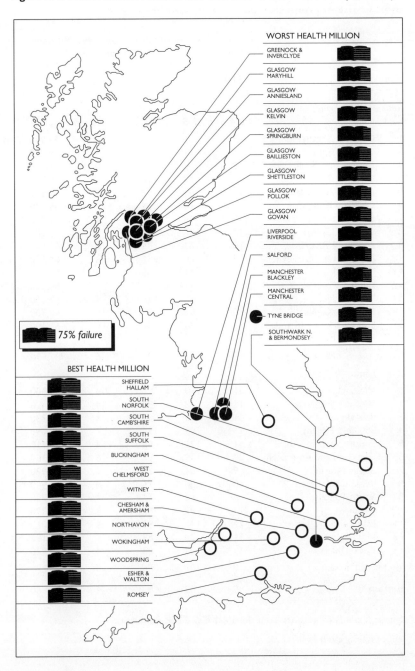

Table 2.6: **Post-school qualifications for constituencies where people are most at risk of premature death in Britain (1991)**

Rank	Name	Higher degrees per 1,000	Degrees per 1,000	Diplomas per 1,000	Qualified unemployed per 1,000	Number of adults
Ratio of 'worst health' to 'best health' areas		**0.4**	**0.5**	**0.5**	**1.5**	**1.0**
1	Glasgow Shettleston	3	31	32	5	45,930
2	Glasgow Springburn	2	17	27	4	49,750
3	Glasgow Maryhill	8	56	38	10	57,180
4	Glasgow Pollok	1	20	38	2	54,830
5	Glasgow Anniesland	10	52	52	4	53,550
6	Glasgow Baillieston	1	14	29	3	53,330
7	Manchester Central	12	44	31	9	66,020
8	Glasgow Govan	12	87	67	8	50,900
9	Liverpool Riverside	10	63	35	10	62,540
10	Manchester Blackley	3	26	31	3	64,120
11	Greenock and Inverclyde	1	41	65	3	49,220
12	Salford	7	37	31	3	59,360
13	Tyne Bridge	4	25	28	4	64,060
14	Glasgow Kelvin	30	167	89	16	45,700
15	Southwark North and Bermondsey	13	75	37	10	61,100
'Worst health' million		*8*	*49*	*41*	*6*	*837,590*
Rank	Name					
1	Wokingham	21	130	96	4	64,500
2	Woodspring	15	78	94	4	66,820
3	Romsey	21	106	94	4	64,330
4	Sheffield Hallam	46	163	120	7	55,090
5	South Cambridgeshire	41	121	95	4	68,110
6	Chesham and Amersham	22	130	91	6	68,360
7	South Norfolk	9	61	70	3	74,980
8	West Chelmsford	10	84	76	4	73,560
9	South Suffolk	8	66	77	3	63,750
10	Witney	17	82	67	3	71,390
11	Esher and Walton	22	131	81	6	75,010
12	Northavon	11	70	89	2	73,190
13	Buckingham	13	103	83	4	59,140
'Best health' million		*19*	*101*	*86*	*4*	*878,230*
Britain		9	62	63	4	41,727,980

Source: Analysis by authors from the 1991 Census of population

Figure 2.5: Post-school qualifications in the extreme areas of Britain (1991)

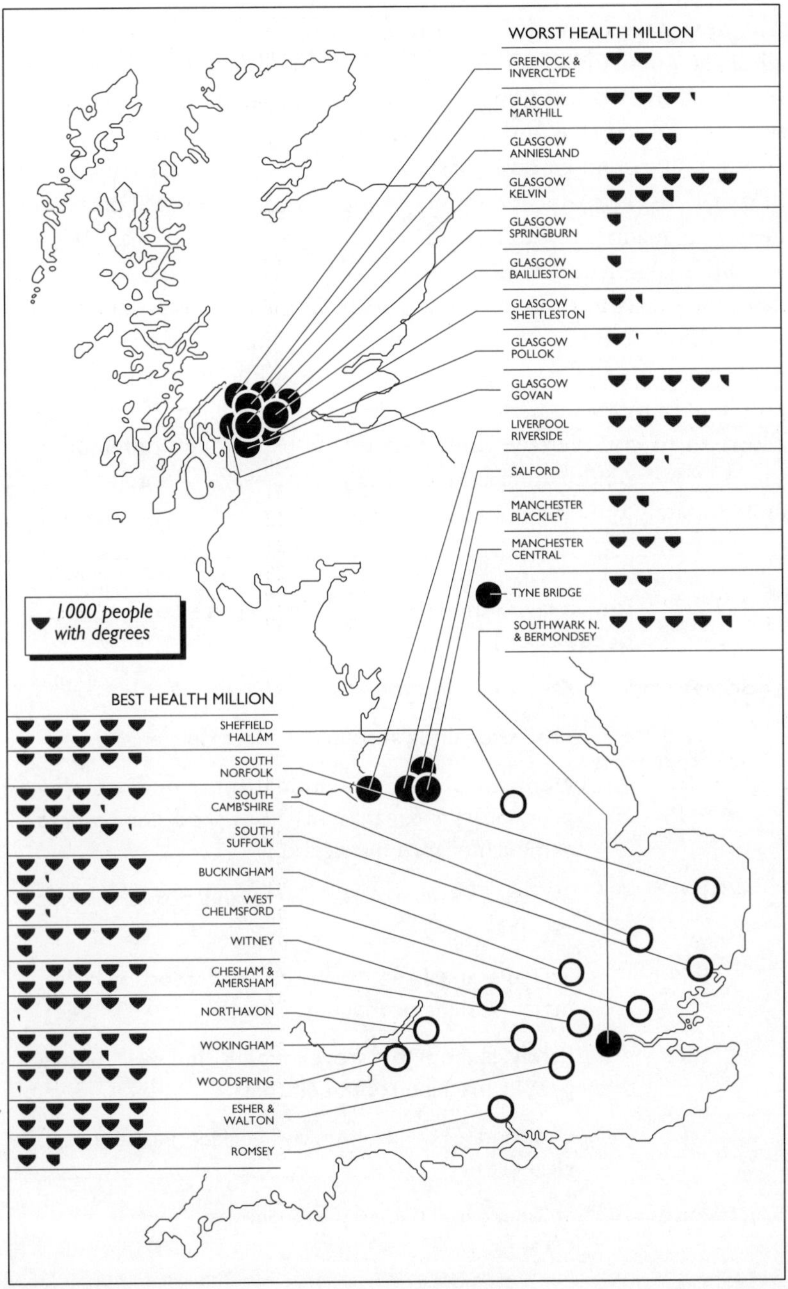

Source: Table 2.6

Occupation – inequalities in working life

The next stage of life after education, for many although by no means all of the population, is the world of work (although these two 'stages' are increasingly overlapping, as many students have to work to pay their way through college, and in a 'flexible' labour market education often continues through working life). The Registrar General's classification of social class is the most commonly used measure of social position in health inequalities research (see Box 2.2). Classes I and II and IV and V are often aggregated, which can serve to hide the true extent of the degree of variation. Table 2.7 uses data from the ONS Longitudinal Study (LS) (see Box 2.3). The LS allows us to look at mortality and life expectancy for all social classes while overcoming the methodological problems of many studies (for more details see Goldblatt, 1990b). It also allows us to consider the full range of life expectancy differences by social class for both men and women. However, as noted above, it unfortunately only includes England and Wales and not Scotland.

Box 2.2: **Registrar General's social class (based on occupation)**

Social class	Occupation type
I	Professional (eg accountant, electronic engineers)
II	Managerial and technical/intermediate (eg proprietors and managers – sales, production, works and maintenance managers)
IIIN	Skilled non-manual (eg clerks and cashiers – not retail)
IIIM	Skilled manual (eg drivers of road goods vehicles, metal working production fitters)
IV	Partly skilled (eg storekeepers and warehouse people, machine tool operators)
V	Unskilled (eg building and civil engineering labourers, cleaners etc)

Source: Bunting (1997)

Table 2.7: Total expectation of life by social class (ONS LS) for men and women, England and Wales (1992-96)

Social class	Men	Women
I	77.7	83.4
II	75.8	81.1
IIIN	75.0	80.4
IIIM	73.5	78.8
IV	72.6	77.7
V	68.2	77.0
All	73.9	79.2

Note: For this analysis social class is as of entry into the study (usually 1971).
Source: Hattersley (1999)

Box 2.3: ONS Longitudinal Study

The ONS Longitudinal Study (LS) is a representative 1% sample of the population of England and Wales containing linked Census data and vital events registrations (births, marriages and deaths) for approximately 500,000 people. The LS was begun in the early 1970s by selecting from those enumerated in the 1971 Census everyone born on any of four particular days. Subsequent samples have been drawn and linked from the 1981 and 1991 Censuses using the LS dates of birth. Population change is reflected by the addition of new sample members born on the LS dates together with the recording of exits via death or emigration. Routinely collected data on mortality, fertility, cancer registration, infant mortality, widow(er)hood and the migration of sample members are linked into the sample using the NHS Central Register (NHSCR) to perform the link.

The LS is a very rich source of data for studying mortality and health by social class. Social class is available for LS members based on the occupational questions in the 1971, 1981 and 1991 Censuses. The 1971 members of the LS cohort were assigned to a social class according to their occupations at the 1971 Census. Similarly, the 1981 cohort were assigned their social class at the 1981 Census. For study members in all cohorts it is thus possible to know how many change social class between Censuses.

Source: Adapted from Bunting (1997)

These latest figures from the LS, for deaths occurring in the period 1992-96, show that the difference in life expectancy between men and women is 5.3 years on average. However, the life expectancy gap by occupational social class is even greater. For men, the difference in life expectancy between social classes I and V is 9.5 years. For women, the difference between social classes I and V is 6.4 years. For both men and women, there is a clear social class gradient to life expectancy. Life expectancy is higher for social class IV than V, IIIM than IV, IIIN than IIIM, and so on, with remarkable consistency. For men, the biggest difference is between social classes IV (partly skilled manual) and social class V (unskilled manual) accounting for 4.4 years of the 9.5 year difference. For women, the biggest difference is between social classes I (professional) and II (managerial and technical/intermediate), accounting for 2.3 of the 6.4 years of difference. As mentioned above, many studies, including ONS reports, often combine social classes I and II and IV and V, and thereby conceal the true extent of the life expectancy difference between the highest and lowest social groups.

We can also consider the difference in life chances by occupational groups by looking at SMRs instead of life expectancy, as in Table 2.8 (see Glossary for an explanation of these and other measures of mortality). The social class gap (for men) is such that for every 100 men who die nationally, 189 men in social class V die, whereas only 66 men in social class I die.

Comparing the 'best health' and 'worst health' areas Table 2.9 shows that 49% more people aged under 65 were in work in the 'best health' areas of Britain compared to the 'worst health' areas, this difference being largely due to differences in unemployment rates and in the number of people who are permanently sick. In addition, those people in work in the 'best health' areas were 57% more likely to have a job in social classes I and II, whereas people in the 'worst health' areas were 72% more likely to be in semi-skilled or unskilled work, or 89% more likely to be in the 'other' category of the armed forces, on training schemes or in otherwise inadequately described occupations.

Table 2.8: SMRs by social class (men aged 20-64), England and Wales (1991-93)

SMR	I	II	III	IV	V	Ratio V:I
1991-93	66	72	113	116	189	**2.9**

Source: Bunting (1997)

Table 2.9: **Social class of people in employment aged over 16 in the extreme areas of Britain in 1991**

Rank Name	All people working	% in I & II	% in III	% in IV & V	% other
Ratio of 'worst health' to 'best health' areas	**0.7**	**0.6**	**1.1**	**1.7**	**1.9**
1 Glasgow Shettleston	18,040	23	46	24	6
2 Glasgow Springburn	20,100	18	46	32	4
3 Glasgow Maryhill	24,72	27	42	26	5
4 Glasgow Pollok	24,600	22	47	26	4
5 Glasgow Anniesland	22,730	29	42	24	5
6 Glasgow Baillieston	23,780	19	50	27	5
7 Manchester Central	25,640	25	39	32	4
8 Glasgow Govan	24,850	41	38	18	3
9 Liverpool Riverside	23,420	30	37	27	7
10 Manchester Blackley	29,450	23	44	30	3
11 Greenock and Inverclyde	24,290	27	41	28	4
12 Salford	27,070	26	43	28	3
13 Tyne Bridge	28,060	19	46	30	5
14 Glasgow Kelvin	22,350	52	31	13	4
15 Southwark North and Bermondsey	29,600	30	42	24	4
'Worst health' million	*368,700*	*27*	*42*	*26*	*4*
Rank Name					
1 Wokingham	45,270	49	37	11	3
2 Woodspring	40,610	42	43	14	1
3 Romsey	39,680	44	38	16	2
4 Sheffield Hallam	30,950	58	30	10	2
5 South Cambridgeshire	42,510	45	37	16	2
6 Chesham and Amersham	43,450	49	38	12	1
7 South Norfolk	44,670	34	44	20	3
8 West Chelmsford	47,480	39	44	16	1
9 South Suffolk	38,440	36	41	20	3
10 Witney	45,890	35	40	18	6
11 Esher and Walton	44,810	49	38	12	1
12 Northavon	48,550	37	45	16	2
13 Buckingham	38,860	44	38	16	2
'Best health' million	*551,170*	*43*	*40*	*15*	*2*
Britain	23,611,270	33	44	21	3

Note: Figures are from the 10% sample, percentages sum to 100.
Source: Analysis by authors of the 1991 Census of population

Figure 2.6: Social classes I & II in the extreme areas of Britain (1991)

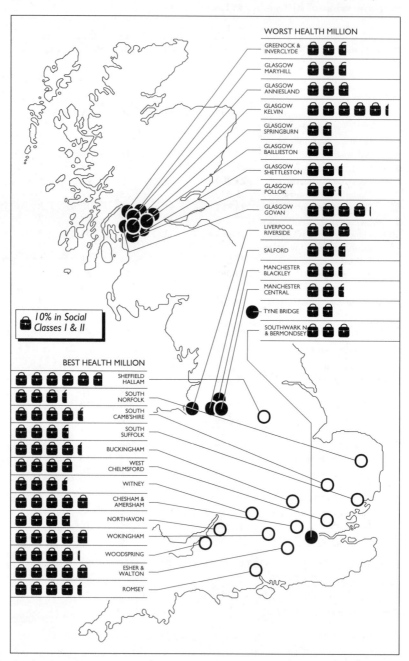

Knowing that there are social class differences in mortality, and that the distribution of social classes is not geographically even, there being more people working in social class I and II occupations in the 'best health' areas and more people in social classes IV and V in the 'worst health' areas, does this social class distribution account for the geographical distribution in mortality? We can answer this question by using the Sample of Anonymised Records (SARs) from the Census and the LS (see Appendix C for more details). For England and Wales as a whole, only 29% of the variation in mortality between local areas can be explained by the geographical distribution of people in different social classes. Figure 2.6 and Table 2.9 illustrate part of the reason for this finding. Although there are about 50% more people in social classes I and II in the 'best health' areas compared to the 'worst health' areas this is not enough of a difference to account for the twofold difference in premature mortality rates. Traditional social class classifications capture some gross inequalities between people's lives in Britain but they do not capture the bulk of social inequalities. For instance, there are more people in classes I and II in both Glasgow Kelvin and Glasgow Govan than in five of the 'best health' constituencies. This does not mean that the former are more prosperous places.

Adults not in work

It is important to remember that the majority of people in Britain do not have a social class allocated to them in the Small Area Statistics (SAS) of the Census (see Glossary). This includes all children aged under 16, all people over retirement age and all people working looking after the home. There are other significant groups of people without a social class: people who have never worked or have not worked for at least 10 years, students and those who are permanently sick. Table 2.10 and Figure 2.7 show how many people are in these situations in the 'worst' and 'best' health areas of Britain and also includes those unemployed but who have had a job in the last 10 years, as these people are excluded from Table 2.9 above. Table 2.10 also shows what proportion of the working population these four groups make up. Overall, in Britain, these groups alone amount to about a quarter of the working age population, but in the 'worst health' areas they are much larger proportion than this. Almost five times as many people have never worked in the 'worst health' areas, while fewer are students (despite the presence of universities near these areas).

Table 2.10: Some groups of people with no current social class aged over 16 in the extreme areas of Britain in 1991

Rank	Name	People who not have worked in last 10 years	Other people who are unemployed	Students	Perma-nently sick	As a % of all people working
Ratio of 'worst health' to 'best health' areas		**4.9**	**2.8**	**0.9**	**4.4**	**3.6**
1	Glasgow Shettleston	2,950	3,834	1,227	5,663	76
2	Glasgow Springburn	3,470	4,684	1,433	5,764	76
3	Glasgow Maryhill	3,630	4,636	2,438	5,897	67
4	Glasgow Pollok	2,810	3,847	1,374	5,116	53
5	Glasgow Anniesland	2,480	3,462	1,770	5,085	56
6	Glasgow Baillieston	3,420	4,327	1,315	6,440	65
7	Manchester Central	4,250	6,762	4,236	6,452	85
8	Glasgow Govan	2,100	3,424	2,210	3,688	46
9	Liverpool Riverside	5,880	5,926	4,118	6,576	96
10	Manchester Blackley	3,240	4,377	2,364	5,440	52
11	Greenock and Inverclyde	1,640	3,357	1,799	4,098	45
12	Salford	2,360	4,372	2,511	5,153	53
13	Tyne Bridge	3,690	5,714	2,267	5,511	61
14	Glasgow Kelvin	1,420	3,112	3,726	3,015	50
15	Southwark North and Bermondsey	3,650	4,665	2,796	3,147	48
	'Worst health' million	*46,990*	*66,499*	*35,584*	*77,045*	*61*
Rank	**Name**					
1	Wokingham	790	1,534	3,402	931	15
2	Woodspring	680	1,864	3,052	1,642	18
3	Romsey	710	1,794	3,080	1,161	17
4	Sheffield Hallam	670	1,670	4,255	1,456	26
5	South Cambridgeshire	550	1,565	3,828	1,456	17
6	Chesham and Amersham	700	1,615	4,014	1,256	17
7	South Norfolk	1,120	1,571	2,523	1,743	16
8	West Chelmsford	710	2,448	2,716	1,215	15
9	South Suffolk	710	1,911	2,483	1,460	17
10	Witney	800	1,896	2,637	1,354	15
11	Esher and Walton	810	1,925	3,746	1,313	17
12	Northavon	900	2,135	3,054	1,598	16
13	Buckingham	510	1,654	3,200	1,094	17
	'Best health' million	*9,660*	*23,582*	*41,990*	*17,679*	*17*
Britain		**919,140**	**1,914,464**	**1,670,918**	**1,795,647**	**27**

Note: People who have not worked in last 10 years figures taken from the 10% sample Census.

Source: Analysis by authors of the 1991 Census of population

Figure 2.7: **Number of people not working in the extreme areas of Britain (1991)**

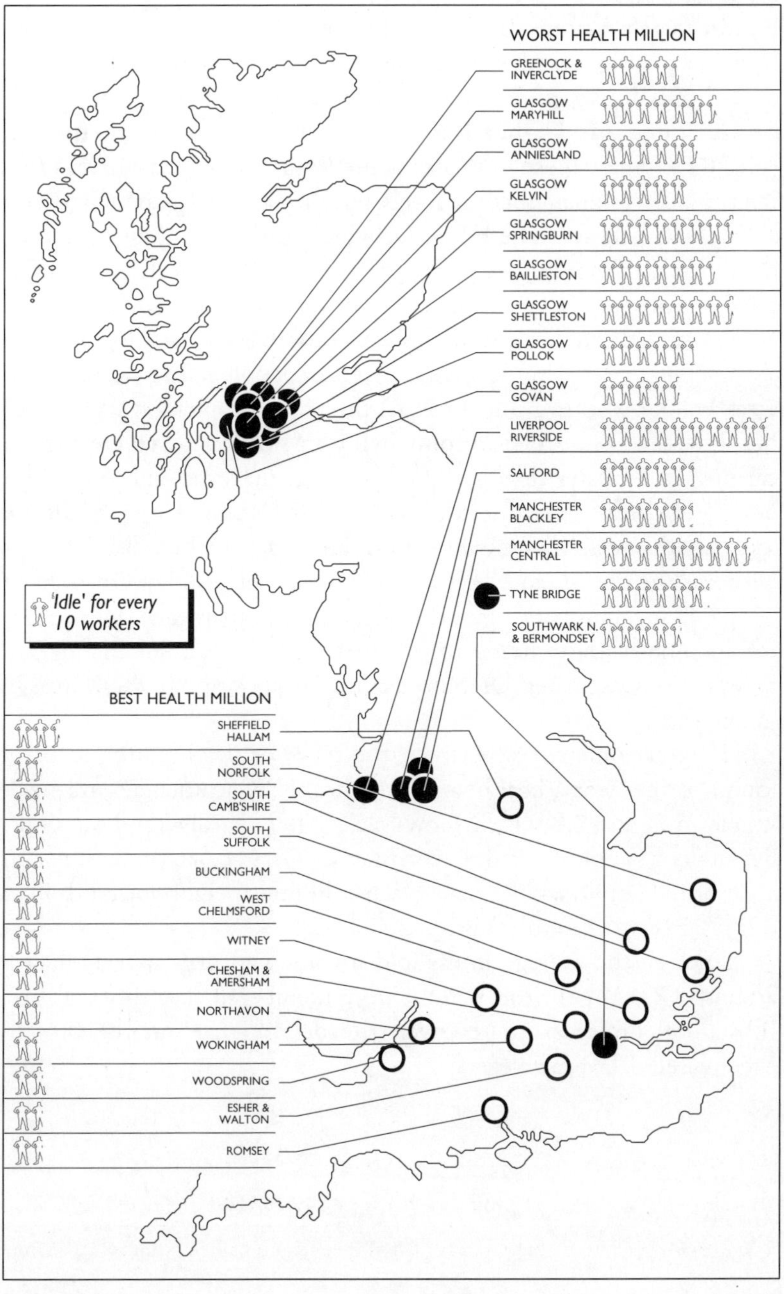

Source: Table 2.10

Income by constituency

Employment status and job titles only give a rough idea of income. Unfortunately income is not asked in the Census but private surveys have been merged with Census data to produce income estimates for households living in small areas which are used by, among other organisations, the Higher Education Funding Council for England (HEFCE). Since these estimates come from commercial surveys they tend to over-estimate income levels, but they are still extremely useful, as Table 2.11 shows. The HEFCE divides Britain into four groups for the purpose of monitoring participation in higher education (HEFCE, 1997). The poorest group is made up of households living in small areas where the median household income is estimated to be below £13,300 per year. Almost three quarters of people in the 'worst health' areas belong to this group, over 12 times the proportion in the 'best health' areas. The richest group, living in small areas where median earnings are greater than £18,000 per year make up only 5% of the population of the 'worst health' areas, almost 10 times fewer than in the 'best health' areas. Income differences are by far the best discriminator between the 'worst' and 'best' areas in terms of health. On average, people living and working in the 'worst health' areas earn only 65% of the income of those living in the 'best health' areas, but this statistic hides the much greater differences in the composition of these areas by income.

The great differences between the types of neighbourhood to be found in the 'worst health' and 'best health' constituencies are made visible in Figure 2.8 which shows clearly how hardly any households live in poor enumeration districts (EDs; see Glossary) in the 'best health' areas of the country, but a majority live in poor neighbourhoods in all of the 15 'worst health' constituencies.

Although the average household income gap may appear small at around £8,000 per year, it must be remembered that this will be a substantial under-estimate given the dependence on the broadly categorised data available.

Table 2.11: Average income and median income bands of households in the extreme areas of Britain by ED (1991)

Rank	Name	Poorest £8.2k-£13.3k	Next poorest £13.4k-£16.1k	Next richest £16.2k-£17.9k	Richest £18.0k-£29.2k	Mean income
Ratio of 'worst health' to 'best health' areas		12.2	1.1	0.2	0.1	0.7
1	Glasgow Shettleston	87	8	4	2	£13,975
2	Glasgow Springburn	89	8	1	1	£13,697
3	Glasgow Maryhill	80	9	4	6	£14,716
4	Glasgow Pollok	77	13	8	2	£14,209
5	Glasgow Anniesland	81	8	4	7	£14,833
6	Glasgow Baillieston	77	7	13	3	£14,277
7	Manchester Central	68	26	1	5	£15,115
8	Glasgow Govan	75	13	3	9	£15,980
9	Liverpool Riverside	63	25	4	8	£15,549
10	Manchester Blackley	60	27	12	2	£15,291
11	Greenock and Inverclyde	66	13	13	8	£15,969
12	Salford	60	27	10	4	£15,897
13	Tyne Bridge	72	20	6	2	£14,763
14	Glasgow Kelvin	67	16	4	13	£17,071
15	Southwark North and Bermondsey	83	9	0	8	£17,030
'Worst health' million		*73*	*17*	*6*	*5*	*£15,101*
Rank	**Name**					
1	Wokingham	2	12	20	66	£24,490
2	Woodspring	4	15	36	45	£22,931
3	Romsey	7	11	38	43	£23,136
4	Sheffield Hallam	10	12	20	58	£24,757
5	South Cambridgeshire	4	13	28	55	£23,864
6	Chesham and Amersham	3	14	20	64	£25,737
7	South Norfolk	5	19	46	30	£21,265
8	West Chelmsford	12	22	36	30	£21,355
9	South Suffolk	11	20	44	25	£21,046
10	Witney	8	21	39	32	£21,298
11	Esher and Walton	5	13	29	53	£25,905
12	Northavon	4	17	45	34	£22,224
13	Buckingham	3	10	33	54	£23,603
'Best health' million		*6*	*16*	*34*	*45*	*£23,153*
Britain		29	26	25	20	£19,460

Note: The 0% of households in quartile 3 in Southwark North and Bermondsey mean that there were no households in quartile 3 EDs in this constituency. Percentages sum to 100% and are of the proportion of households living in Census EDs in each quartile of the country divided by income. Mean income is of households from commercial surveys.

Source: Analysis by authors from estimates published by HEFCE (1997)

Figure 2.8: Proportion of families in poor neighbourhoods in the extreme areas of Britain (1991)

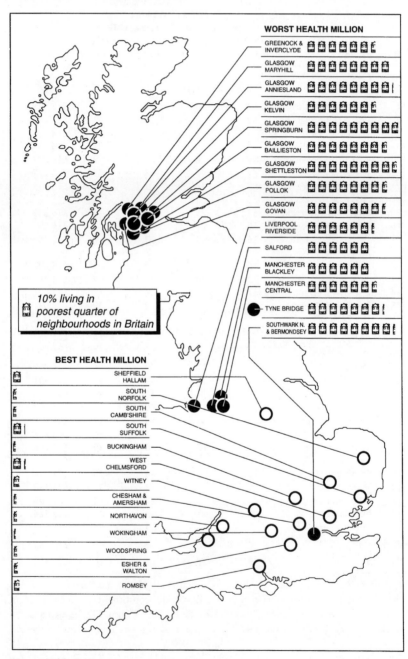

Source: Table 2.11

We have one alternative source of income estimates that we can use to help validate the above findings. This is derived from the occupational data collected in the Census and refers to individuals rather than households and wards rather than EDs (see Glossary for definitions of geographical units). Table 2.12 shows average income calculated from the detailed occupational status and employment categories of adults in the 1991 Census, adjusted for differential average pay rates between men and women, with occupational income coming from the *New Earnings* survey (1991). These data are only available at ward level and so the results differ from those above, but in terms of proportions with low and high incomes they show more extreme differences between these two sets of constituencies as they grade areas more finely. People are more than 100 times more likely to be living in wards containing the poorest quartile of the population in the 'worst health' constituencies. In Figure 2.9 the average incomes for working people in these areas are mapped to illustrate that the mean differences between areas are only of the order of a few thousand pounds. Two thirds of adults living in the 'best health' constituencies in the country live in wards in the highest quartile of incomes, whereas 70% of adults living in the 'worst health' constituencies live in wards which contain the quarter of the population with the lowest average ward incomes. However, it should be noted that a much lower proportion of people are working in the 'worst health' areas, and hence these 'average incomes' are somewhat misleading.

If we consider the poorest and richest 10% of wards in Britain by average adult incomes we see that the differences in terms of income distribution between these areas are even more extreme. Just over half of all adults in the 'worst health' constituencies live in wards that fall into the category of the poorest 10% of wards in the country. This poorest tenth has average incomes that are below £9,600 per year. Note that this only includes adults in work or receiving unemployment benefit or working on a government scheme. Children and adults not in the workforce (such as single parents, the early retired and the permanently sick) are not included and there are more people being counted in the richest areas. Most importantly, nobody who lives in the richest million population areas lives in a ward that is in the poorest 10% of wards in Britain.

Table 2.12: **Extreme income bands of adults in the workforce in the extreme areas of Britain by ward (1991)**

Rank Name	Prop-ortion in poorest 10% £5.8k-£9.6k	Prop-ortion in poorest 25% £5.8k-10.6k	Prop-ortion in richest 25% £12.7k-17.0k	Prop-ortion in richest 25% £13.6k-£17.0k	Mean income (1991 prices)
Ratio of 'worst health' to 'best health' areas	na	131.2	0.13	0.12	0.75
1 Glasgow Shettleston	61	68	0	0	£9,009
2 Glasgow Springburn	55	61	8	0	£9,462
3 Glasgow Maryhill	68	91	9	9	£9,347
4 Glasgow Pollok	37	84	0	0	£9,448
5 Glasgow Anniesland	57	69	31	16	£10,380
6 Glasgow Baillieston	46	8	8	0	£9,457
7 Manchester Central	84	84	0	0	£8,959
8 Glasgow Govan	30	41	32	6	£11,356
9 Liverpool Riverside	66	81	0	0	£8,794
10 Manchester Blackley	52	86	0	0	£9,640
11 Greenock and Inverclyde	67	67	11	0	£10,007
12 Salford	46	68	0	0	£10,072
13 Tyne Bridge	74	100	0	0	£8,794
14 Glasgow Kelvin	7	16	50	34	£12,724
15 Southwark North and Bermondsey	18	42	0	0	£10,825
'Worst health' million	52	70	9	4	£9,837
Rank Name					
1 Wokingham	0	0	98	77	£14,127
2 Woodspring	0	0	58	16	£12,853
3 Romsey	0	0	63	19	£13,087
4 Sheffield Hallam	0	0	100	74	£14,078
5 South Cambridgeshire	0	0	88	40	£13,323
6 Chesham and Amersham	0	0	88	42	£13,651
7 South Norfolk	0	4	17	5	£12,144
8 West Chelmsford	0	0	59	14	£12,986
9 South Suffolk	0	0	47	9	£12,386
10 Witney	0	1	49	4	£12,582
11 Esher and Walton	0	0	82	70	£14,001
12 Northavon	0	2	46	12	£12,433
13 Buckingham	0	0	76	23	£13,247
'Best health' million	0	1	66	30	£13,127
Britain	10	25	25	10	£11,619

Note: Mean income estimates are for adults in work or unemployed. The proportions are of all adults in each constituency, who live in wards in the richest and poorest 10% and 25% in the country.

Source: Analysis by authors based on the 1991 Census of populations and the 1991 *New Earnings* survey

***Figure 2.9:* Mean income of adults in the workforce in the extreme areas of Britain (1991)**

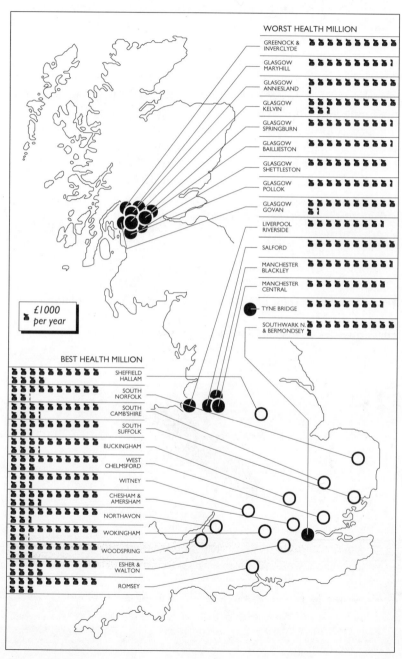

Source: Table 2.12

Poverty, deprivation and health

We can also look at this connection between health and income by again considering poverty, as in the section referring to children above (see Table 2.4). Figure 2.10 shows how closely related premature mortality and poverty are, as measured by the *Breadline Britain* index. The correlation coefficient for this relationship is such that r = 0.85 (see Glossary). The ecological relationship — that is, at the area rather than individual level — between high rates of poverty in an area and high rates of mortality is thus extremely close. This is the closest single ecological relationship there is to explain differences in premature mortality in Britain. Around two thirds of the variation in death rates between areas can be explained by the level of poverty in these areas. However, to be certain that the relationship is not an 'ecological fallacy' — that it really is poverty that is leading to ill-health and not, for instance, that living next door to poor households leads to poor health — we need to consider the individual level data on poverty and illness in Britain, and these are examined in Chapter 3.

Figure 2.10: **Scatterplot of SMR for deaths under 65 and % of households living in poverty (*Breadline Britain* index), for parliamentary constituencies, Britain (1991-95)**

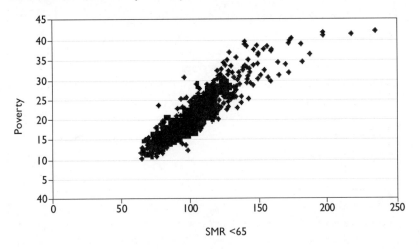

Source: Analysis by authors; see Appendix A for constituency data

Unemployment – inequalities in the labour market

Those who are unemployed have, in the main, low incomes, but unemployment also has independent effects on health and so needs separate consideration here. There is evidence that all people who experience unemployment for more than a short period of time have an increased risk of adverse health outcomes. Morris and colleagues (1994) studied more than 6,000 men aged 40-59 over a five-year period, comparing those who had experienced some unemployment over that time with those who had retired and those who were continuously employed. Over the five-year period 96% of those in work survived, compared to only 91% of those who experienced unemployment. They found that compared to those who had been in continuous employment, those who had been unemployed at some point over the five-year study period were almost twice as likely to die in any year. This effect was found when factors such as social class and health-related behaviours (smoking, alcohol consumption and body weight) and also health status at the beginning of the five years had been taken into account. Those who experienced unemployment were thus not more likely to die just because they smoked more, nor because they were more likely to be in an unskilled job or because they were ill at the start of the five-year period. Instead, it appears that unemployment itself has a detrimental effect upon health.

Why is unemployment detrimental to health? Unemployment usually brings financial hardship, itself associated with poorer health; but it can also lead to social isolation and loss of self-esteem. There are a number of benefits which people derive from work, in addition to the financial reward: having a structure and purpose to the day, self-respect, the respect of others, physical and mental activity, use of skills, interpersonal contact and social status (Bartley, 1994). The unemployed have been found to have higher rates of depression and anxiety and lower levels of psychological well-being (Bartley, 1994). Montgomery et al (1999) found unemployment to be a risk factor for psychological symptoms of depression requiring medical attention, even in those men who did not have any history of psychological problems. Another recent study has reported that those who had experienced unemployment were more than twice as likely to commit suicide than were people who had not experienced unemployment (Lewis and Sloggett, 1998). Crucially, it has also been found that the anticipation of job loss or job insecurity affects health – Ferrie and colleagues (1995, 1998) have found that the anticipation of possible job loss produces a significant deterioration in self-reported health and various objective health indicators relative to those in secure employment.

As we have already observed, unemployment is extremely unevenly distributed spatially. As Table 2.13 shows, unemployment rates of those men aged 16-64 in the 'worst health' areas stood at 20% of all men in 1991, four times more than the rate in the 'best health' areas and twice the national average. A further 12% of men in the 'worst health' areas were permanently sick, more than five times higher than the rate in the 'best health' areas. Permanent sickness is often a hidden form of unemployment, and this is partly reflected in the very high rates of sickness in these areas. Other forms of economic inactivity (principally being on a government scheme) are also three times more common in the 'worst health' areas. Early retirement, however, is very slightly more common in the better off areas, possibly a reflection of the prevalence of private pension schemes. It is difficult to know, however, the extent to which early retirement is due to choice (and accompanied by private pension provision) and how much is related to ill-health and is thus enforced.

The huge disparity in the proportion of men not working between our two sets of areas of Britain is shown starkly in Figure 2.11. There is some variation within the two groups of constituencies, but this is minimal when compared to the differences between the 'worst health' and 'best health' areas. Clearly being out of work in such large numbers damages the health of men of working age in these places.

The geographical gap for women's participation in the labour market (Table 2.14) is not as wide as for men because in both the 'best health' and 'worst health' areas about a quarter of women aged 16-65 are working/looking after the home and children. We have included women aged 60-64 in the table to make these figures comparable with the mortality rates in this book, but this increases the overall proportion not in work as the official retirement age for women is still 60 years of age. However, in the 'worst health' areas in Britain women are still twice as likely to be either unemployed or permanently sick compared to women in the 'best health' areas. Again there is little difference between the rates of early retirement for these areas. Figure 2.12 shows that the geographical differences in employment for women between the two sets of areas are not as great as for men.

Table 2.13: **Percentage unemployed, permanently sick and inactive, for men aged 16-64 in the extreme areas of Britain (1991)**

Rank	Name	Unem-ployed	Perm sick	Early retired	Other	Total
Ratio of 'worst health' to 'best health' areas		**3.9**	**5.2**	**0.9**	**3.3**	**3.4**
I	Glasgow Shettleston	22.9	16.0	2.6	4.4	45.8
2	Glasgow Springburn	25.0	15.2	2.5	4.4	47.2
3	Glasgow Maryhill	21.6	12.8	2.0	4.4	40.8
4	Glasgow Pollok	19.8	12.0	2.1	4.4	38.3
5	Glasgow Anniesland	18.5	13.1	2.5	3.9	38.0
6	Glasgow Baillieston	21.0	14.1	1.8	4.6	41.6
7	Manchester Central	23.6	11.8	2.3	3.7	41.5
8	Glasgow Govan	16.1	8.9	1.8	3.3	30.0
9	Liverpool Riverside	26.3	12.0	2.3	4.5	45.0
10	Manchester Blackley	18.8	10.9	2.2	2.9	34.8
11	Greenock and Inverclyde	14.9	10.8	2.9	3.1	31.6
12	Salford	18.5	11.1	2.0	2.5	34.0
13	Tyne Bridge	22.2	11.8	2.2	4.1	40.4
14	Glasgow Kelvin	14.0	8.3	2.0	3.1	27.4
15	Southwark North and Bermondsey	18.5	5.9	1.8	2.8	29.0
'Worst health' million		*20.3*	*11.5*	*2.2*	*3.7*	*37.7*
Rank	**Name**					
I	Wokingham	4.4	1.3	1.8	1.0	8.5
2	Woodspring	5.5	2.6	3.6	1.0	12.7
3	Romsey	5.7	2.0	2.9	1.1	11.7
4	Sheffield Hallam	6.1	3.1	3.2	1.5	14.0
5	South Cambridgeshire	4.4	2.3	2.0	0.8	9.5
6	Chesham and Amersham	4.7	1.9	2.6	0.8	10.0
7	South Norfolk	5.2	2.9	2.4	1.3	11.8
8	West Chelmsford	6.1	2.0	1.9	1.0	11.1
9	South Suffolk	6.1	2.6	2.6	1.1	12.3
10	Witney	5.0	2.2	1.8	1.2	10.2
11	Esher and Walton	5.4	1.7	2.7	0.9	10.7
12	Northavon	5.3	2.4	2.2	1.5	11.3
13	Buckingham	4.8	1.9	2.0	1.4	10.1
'Best health' million		*5.3*	*2.2*	*2.4*	*1.1*	*11.0*
Britain		9.8	5.3	2.5	2.1	19.6

Note: 'Other' refers to those on government schemes or otherwise not in work, 'Total' is all not employed or in education.

Source: Analysis by authors of the 1991 Census of populations

Unemployed	Unemployed as a % of all men aged 16-64
Perm sick	% of all men permanently sick aged 16-64
Early retired	% of all men retired aged 16-64
Other	All other men not working but of working age

Figure 2.11: Men aged 16-64 not working in the extreme areas of Britain (1991)

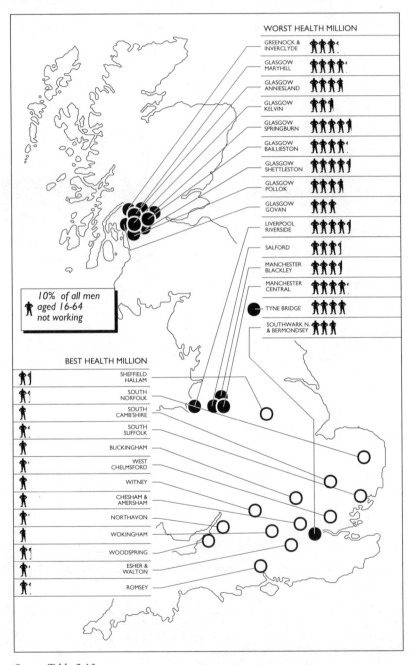

Source: Table 2.13

Table 2.14: **Percentage unemployed, permanently sick and inactive, for women aged 16-64 in the extreme areas of Britain (1991)**

Rank Name		Unemployed	Perm sick	Early retired	Other	Total
Ratio of 'worst health' to 'best health' areas		**3.2**	**4.9**	**1.4**	**1.1**	**1.5**
1	Glasgow Shettleston	9.2	10.8	6.7	26.7	53.5
2	Glasgow Springburn	10.6	9.9	6.5	26.7	53.8
3	Glasgow Maryhill	8.6	9.0	5.4	25.6	48.6
4	Glasgow Pollok	7.2	8.3	6.4	27.2	49.0
5	Glasgow Anniesland	7.3	8.6	6.9	24.6	47.4
6	Glasgow Baillieston	8.5	10.7	5.0	30.2	54.5
7	Manchester Central	10.4	7.7	5.3	29.3	52.6
8	Glasgow Govan	6.9	6.0	5.6	23.1	41.6
9	Liverpool Riverside	12.0	8.0	4.8	27.6	52.3
10	Manchester Blackley	7.3	6.9	6.1	26.9	47.3
11	Greenock and Inverclyde	6.2	6.1	5.9	23.7	41.9
12	Salford	7.1	7.7	5.8	24.4	45.0
13	Tyne Bridge	8.3	6.5	5.3	29.1	49.2
14	Glasgow Kelvin	6.0	5.7	5.4	15.1	32.1
15	Southwark North and Bermondsey	9.4	4.1	4.6	23.7	41.8
'Worst health' million		*8.4*	*7.7*	*5.7*	*25.9*	*47.6*
Rank Name						
1	Wokingham	2.4	1.1	3.2	21.2	27.9
2	Woodspring	2.5	1.9	4.6	22.2	31.1
3	Romsey	2.5	1.4	4.4	23.3	31.6
4	Sheffield Hallam	2.9	2.1	6.1	18.8	29.9
5	South Cambridgeshire	2.2	1.7	3.6	20.7	28.2
6	Chesham and Amersham	2.5	1.5	3.8	23.7	31.5
7	South Norfolk	2.4	1.8	5.0	24.9	34.2
8	West Chelmsford	3.1	1.4	4.0	22.6	31.2
9	South Suffolk	2.8	1.7	4.9	24.8	34.3
10	Witney	2.6	1.4	3.7	22.4	30.0
11	Esher and Walton	2.8	1.5	3.9	26.1	34.3
12	Northavon	2.6	1.7	3.6	21.7	29.6
13	Buckingham	2.7	1.2	3.8	23.0	30.7
'Best health' million		*2.6*	*1.6*	*4.1*	*22.8*	*31.1*
Britain		**4.4**	**3.5**	**5.1**	**23.6**	**36.6**

Note: 'Other' refers to those on government schemes or otherwise not in work; 'Total' is all not employed or in education.

Source: Analysis by authors of the 1991 Census of populations

Unemployed	Unemployed as a % of all women aged 16-64
Perm sick	% of all women permanently sick aged 16-64
Early retired	% of all women retired aged 16-64
Other	All other women not working but of working age

Figure 2.12: Women aged 16-64 not working in the extreme areas of Britain (1991)

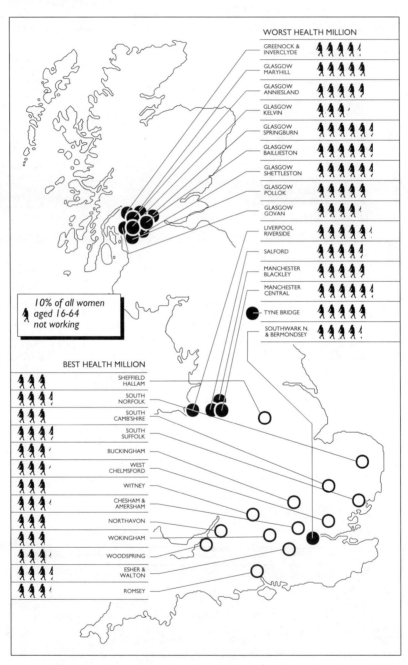

Source: Table 2.14

Inequalities in illness

The most direct precursor to premature death in 1990s Britain is illness. There are several studies which have found that illness is more prevalent in groups of people living in more deprived areas. For example, the Somerset and Avon survey of health (Eachus et al, 1996) studied various indicators of self-reported health among over 28,000 individuals aged over 35 and related these health measures to Townsend deprivation scores (which take into account unemployment, car access, owner-occupation and overcrowded households in the areas within which people live). The results show that material deprivation in the local community is strongly linked with many common diseases – including heart attacks, depression and stroke; the diseases most strongly linked to deprivation were bronchitis and emphysema.

Data from the Health Education Monitoring Survey (Hansbro et al, 1997) – which surveyed 4,600 adults aged 16-74 in England – also reported a socio-economic gradient in self-reported health. This study reported age-standardised ratios for overall self-reported health; these can be interpreted like SMRs – the average for all men is 100. The ratio of self-reported 'very good' or 'good' health was 91 for social classes IV and V compared to 106 for classes I and II. Similar ratios are reported for limiting long-term illness (LLTI) by social class, from the same survey.

In 1991 a Census question on LLTI was asked for the first time. For residents in Britain aged under 65, 74 per 1,000, or 7.4%, said they suffered from such an illness. However, if we look at the LLTI rates in the constituencies with the highest mortality rates (the 'worst health' areas) we see that these range from 88 per 1,000 to 161 per 1,000 people aged under 65 (see Table 2.15 and Figure 2.13). An age-sex-standardised illness ratio can be calculated, a concept similar to the SMR, and this shows that the million people in the 'worst health' constituencies were 2.8 times more likely to report being ill in 1991 than were the million living in the 'best health' constituencies. Given this wide health gap it is hardly surprising that people in the 'worst health' constituencies were 2.6 times more likely to subsequently die young in the five years following the Census than those in the 'best health' constituencies (see Table 2.1). The astute reader will note that in each group there are just under a million residents actually reporting. That is mainly because this table excludes those who did not complete the Census form in 1991, those who were in institutions and those who were born after 1991. The final column refers to 'avoidable' illness, the percentage of illness that would not have occurred if the 'worst health' areas had the illness rate of the 'best health' areas. Nearly two thirds of illness is 'avoidable' by this definition.

Table 2.15: **Limiting long-term illness rates for constituencies where people are most and least at risk of premature death in Britain (1991)**

Rank	Name	Obs<65	Rate/1,000	SIR<65	Res<65	Avoidable
	Ratio of 'worst health' to 'best health' areas	**2.7**	**2.7**	**2.8**	**1.0**	
1	Glasgow Shettleston	7,880	161	208	48,920	67%
2	Glasgow Springburn	8,494	155	202	54,875	67%
3	Glasgow Maryhill	8,686	136	188	63,660	64%
4	Glasgow Pollok	7,930	130	173	60,821	61%
5	Glasgow Anniesland	7,366	135	176	54,397	62%
6	Glasgow Baillieston	8,900	138	195	64,333	65%
7	Manchester Central	10,603	128	189	82,914	64%
8	Glasgow Govan	5,501	99	142	55,514	52%
9	Liverpool Riverside	9,268	128	181	72,428	63%
10	Manchester Blackley	8,591	115	164	74,406	59%
11	Greenock and Inverclyde	5,487	101	134	54,194	49%
12	Salford	7,798	118	165	66,205	59%
13	Tyne Bridge	8,625	119	172	72,213	61%
14	Glasgow Kelvin	4,218	93	127	45,199	46%
15	Southwark North and Bermondsey	6,365	88	128	72,557	47%
	'Worst health' million	*115,712*	*123*	*170*	*942,636*	*60%*
Rank	**Name**	**Obs<65**	**Rate/1000**	**SIR<65**	**Res<65**	
1	Wokingham	2,805	36	51	78,902	
2	Woodspring	3,387	46	60	73,189	
3	Romsey	3,147	44	58	70,747	
4	Sheffield Hallam	2,974	53	68	55,938	
5	South Cambridgeshire	3,385	45	60	75,950	
6	Chesham and Amersham	3,055	40	51	76,440	
7	South Norfolk	4,172	53	68	78,314	
8	West Chelmsford	3,744	45	64	82,532	
9	South Suffolk	3,506	51	67	68,878	
10	Witney	3,641	45	63	80,256	
11	Esher and Walton	3,256	41	54	79,990	
12	Northavon	3,768	44	60	85,907	
13	Buckingham	2,850	42	57	68,143	
	'Best health' million	*43,690*	*45*	*60*	*975,186*	
Britain		**3,394,220**	**74**	**100**	**46,049,455**	

Source: Analysis by authors of the 1991 Census of population

Obs<65	Number of people under 65 reporting a LLTI
Rate/1,000	Rate of illness per 1,000 people
SIR<65	Standardised Illness Ratio for under 65s
Res<65	Number of people resident in the constituency under the age of 65
Avoidable	% of illness which would not have occurred if the 'worst illness' areas had the death rate of the 'best health' areas

Figure 2.13: **Standardised limiting long-term illness rates under 65 in the extreme areas of Britain (1991)**

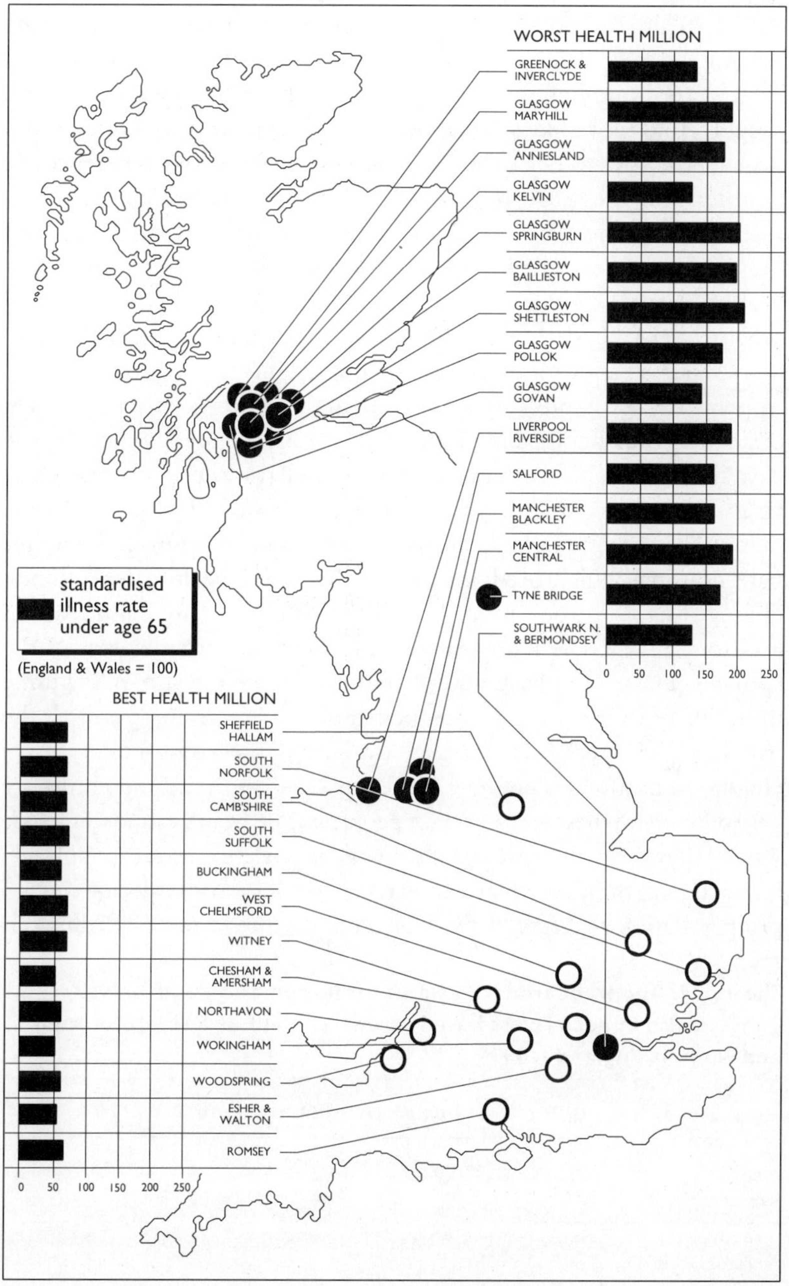

WORST HEALTH MILLION

GREENOCK & INVERCLYDE
GLASGOW MARYHILL
GLASGOW ANNIESLAND
GLASGOW KELVIN
GLASGOW SPRINGBURN
GLASGOW BAILLIESTON
GLASGOW SHETTLESTON
GLASGOW POLLOK
GLASGOW GOVAN
LIVERPOOL RIVERSIDE
SALFORD
MANCHESTER BLACKLEY
MANCHESTER CENTRAL
TYNE BRIDGE
SOUTHWARK N. & BERMONDSEY

0   50   100 150 200 250

standardised illness rate under age 65

(England & Wales = 100)

BEST HEALTH MILLION

SHEFFIELD HALLAM
SOUTH NORFOLK
SOUTH CAMB'SHIRE
SOUTH SUFFOLK
BUCKINGHAM
WEST CHELMSFORD
WITNEY
CHESHAM & AMERSHAM
NORTHAVON
WOKINGHAM
WOODSPRING
ESHER & WALTON
ROMSEY

0   50 100 150 200 250

Source: Table 2.15

53

The morbidity health gap reported above between the 'best health' and 'worst health' areas is again partly a reflection of the different social class compositions of these areas, but again, as for mortality inequalities, this is only a small part of the explanation as to why people living in the extreme areas of Britain should experience such different life chances. Table 2.16 shows how men and women in the higher social classes are roughly 16% more likely to report having 'good' or 'very good' health than in the lower social classes. The two to threefold differences in morbidity by area reported above can thus not be accounted for by social class at one point in time, even if all people living in the 'best health' areas were in the highest classes and all those living in the 'worst health' areas were in the lowest classes. Social class only explains a small proportion of the spatial patterns of inequalities in illness, partly because, as we reported above, most people are not assigned a social class (also see Appendix C). More importantly, being healthy is often a hidden prerequisite for being able to afford to live in the areas where people have the best health (for instance, you often have to be well enough to be in work to be able to pay the mortgage required to have a home there). Similarly, being sick, or having been sick, increases eligibility for state housing, which predominates in the 'worst health' areas. Illness rates also have a strong influence on the patterns of migration which lead to many people living in (or leaving) these extreme areas of the country. Those who have never been seriously ill are very many times more likely to be living in the 'best health' areas as compared to the 'worst health' areas of Britain. However, as the large differences in childhood death rates presented in Table 2.2 show, health outcomes are very different in these areas even for people whose health cannot influence where they live. Fundamentally, living in an area where people are likely to have poor health, because living conditions are inferior and job prospects are low, are all likely to affect a person's chances of falling ill.

Table 2.16: **Age-standardised ratios for self-reported 'good' or 'very good' health by social class based on own current or last job, for men and women, England (1991)**

	I/II	IIIN	IIIM	IV/V
Men	106	99	98	91
Women	107	102	94	92

Source: Hansbro et al (1997)

To demonstrate how much of the inequalities in illness between the 'best health' and 'worst health' areas of Britain are caused by areal difference, not social class, we have calculated from the 1991 Census the proportion of all people who are adults with a LLTI by area type and according to the socio-economic group of their head of household. This is shown in Table 2.17. The categories used here are socio-economic groups rather than social classes (see Glossary), and these are used because the Census results for LLTI by social class for areas are not released.

Table 2.17: **Limiting long-term illness by socio-economic group, men and women, in the extreme areas of Britain (1991)**

	Britain	'Worst health' areas	'Best health' areas	Ratio
		% with LLTI		
Total	11.8	16.7	8.5	2.0
Economically inactive (eg retired, looking after home)	30.6	31.7	27.1	1.2
Skilled manual workers (eg builder, baker, driver)	16.6	22.4	16.2	1.4
Unskilled manual workers (eg road sweeper)	6.5	7.2	7.6	0.9
Inadequately described or not working for 10 years	5.8	7.2	4.4	1.6
Farmers – own account (has only family employees)	5.7	-	2.5	-
Semi-skilled manual workers (eg care assistant)	5.6	6.1	4.7	1.3
Farmers – employers and managers (who own/rent)	4.6	-	2.6	-
Personal service workers (eg chef, waiter/ess)	4.3	4.3	4.3	1.0
Agricultural workers (eg forester, fishing worker)	4.3	7.8	5.8	1.4
Forepersons and supervisors – manual (eg storekeeper)	4.3	5.3	4.2	1.3
Junior non-manual workers (eg check-out operator)	4.1	4.9	3.6	1.4
Self employed non-professionals without employees	4.0	5.6	3.1	1.8
Forepersons and supervisors – non-manual (eg clerk)	3.7	3.7	1.4	2.7
Ancillary workers and artists (eg teacher, nurse)	3.5	4.1	2.9	1.4
Employers and managers in small establishments	3.1	4.1	2.4	1.7
Professional workers (eg architect) self-employed	3.0	2.4	2.4	1.0
Professional workers (eg solicitor) – employees	2.7	3.2	2.6	1.3
Employers and managers in large establishments	2.7	3.2	2.2	1.5
Members of armed forces (all ranks and occupations)	1.8	3.9	1.8	2.2
Active, never worked	1.2	3.6	0.5	6.9

Note: The rates for those who are 'Active, never worked' are relatively low as these people are generally young.

Source: Analysis by authors of the 1991 Census of population

Table 2.17 shows that overall, 11.8% of all people in Britain are adults with a LLTI, but the rate is twice as high (16.7%) in the 'worst health' areas compared to the 'best health' areas (8.5%). The bulk of this difference is due to differences between people who are in the workforce as people in households headed by economically inactive people are only 17% more likely to be suffering from an illness in the 'worst health' areas. Skilled manual workers are the socio-economic group most likely to be ill in Britain, and 39% more report a LLTI in the 'worst health' areas compared to the 'best health' areas. The socio-economic group with the second highest prevalence of LLTI is unskilled manual workers, but for them there is no difference in rates between the 'best health' and 'worst health' areas. The biggest gap between the two sets of areas is for people who have never worked. Of these, those living in the 'worst health' areas of Britain are seven times more likely to report having a LLTI. Of all the socio-economic groups shown in the table, in 14 cases people living in the 'worst health' areas are more than 25% more likely to be ill – despite doing the same kinds of work. In two cases a comparison cannot be made, due to the low prevalence of farmers living in the 'worst health' areas. And in three cases there is no difference for people working in the two sets of areas (unskilled manual workers, eg road sweeper; personal service workers, eg chef, waiter/waitress; professional workers, eg architect).

Wealth – houses and car ownership

So far we have considered employment and occupational status as well as income and poverty in relation to the geography of health in Britain. Another important facet of a person's socio-economic position is wealth. There are very few reliable sources of data on the wealth of individuals in Britain, and so researchers tend to refer to housing tenure and car ownership as indicators of wealth.

Various studies have reported an association between health and housing tenure – whether people own or rent their homes. In a recent study, Filakti and Fox (1995) found that the death rates of men living in privately rented accommodation were 38% higher than those for owner-occupiers (those who own their home outright or who have a mortgage) whereas death rates for people renting their homes from local authorities (council or social housing) were 62% higher. For women, the differences were 38% and 44% respectively. We can see tenure as being a reflection of social class and area of residence, but also of individual wealth too.

Thus a relatively wealthy professor living in a poor area is much more likely to own his or her home than are his or her neighbours.

We should also consider those who do not have a home in the traditional sense and thus cannot be classified to a housing tenure category – the homeless. While housing policy in the last two decades in Britain has led to a dramatic increase in the number of owner–occupiers, rising from 10 million owner–occupiers in 1971 to 16 million in 1993, there has also been a striking increase in the number of homeless people (Dorling, 1995). There is much evidence that the homeless suffer much higher rates of illness than the general population (Bines, 1994), and that they have problems in gaining access to healthcare services (Fisher and Collins, 1993). There is also evidence that they have very high death rates when compared to the general population – rough sleepers in London have been found to have death rates 25 times those of the general population (Shaw and Dorling, 1998).

Access to a car – which is a fairly weak indicator of access to wealth and perhaps better seen as an indicator of available income (Goldblatt, 1990a) – is also often used in studies of health as, like tenure, car access is routinely included in national Censuses. Smith and Harding (1997) present data on the LS cohort, following up those from the 1971 Census over 21 years to 1992. Table 2.18 shows the difference in SMRs by housing tenure within social class and car ownership categories. From this we can see that the lowest SMRs are among those in non–manual occupations with access to a car and in owner–occupied homes. There is a clear relationship between mortality and car access and mortality and housing tenure. However, the relationship with class is less clear. Those in non–manual social classes without access to a car and living in local authority housing have SMRs almost as high as those in manual social classes without access to a car and living in local authority housing. Again, occupational social class may not be the best way in which groups of the population can be divided in terms of their health chances.

Both housing tenure and car access can be seen as indirect indicators of household assets and the long-term command over resources (Smith and Harding, 1997), but it is important to remember that both are also indicators of the type of area in which people live. Houses of the same tenure tend to be clustered in certain areas. In many parts of the country, for instance, it is now impossible to live in a council house, as they have all been either sold to owner–occupiers or transferred to housing association tenure. There are also spatial aspects to car ownership. In many rural areas access to a car is a necessity, whereas for those living in urban areas with good public transport it is less essential.

Indicators of wealth, including measures based on housing, show extreme differences between the two sets of areas we have been following (see Table 2.19). The 'best health' areas have nine times more households with access to three or more cars – and in total almost three times as many cars. These areas also have more than six times as many households with seven or more rooms in their home and 25% more rooms in total, and that is despite having a smaller total number of households. Rooms counted in the Census include rooms that a household has for its own use which are either living rooms, bedrooms, kitchens at least 2 metres wide, and any other rooms other than small kitchens, bathrooms or toilets. It is likely that in the 'best health' areas the rooms were larger, lighter and less damp, and that the cars were newer and more expensive. The Census, however, does not provide statistics on the value of goods and property owned, just the numbers. Even the crude data available are telling enough. Figure 2.14 illustrates that at the extremes there are very high inequalities in access to these basic assets.

Table 2.18: SMRs, by social class, access to cars and housing tenure at the 1971 Census, women and men, all causes, England and Wales (1971-92)

	Age at death 45-64	
	Women	Men
Non-manual social class		
Car		
Owner-occupied	70	72
Privately rented	82	83
Local authority	93	96
No car		
Owner-occupied	91	99
Privately rented	105	129
Local authority	125	120
Manual social class		
Car		
Owner-occupied	85	82
Privately rented	100	93
Local authority	101	104
No car		
Owner-occupied	99	101
Privately rented	128	132
Local authority	131	126

Note: England and Wales = 100.

Source: Adapted from Smith and Harding (1997)

Table 2.19: **Wealth indicators for households in the extreme areas of Britain (1991)**

Rank	Name	House-holds with 3+ cars	Total number of cars	House-holds owning 7+ rooms	Total rooms in the area	House-holds
Ratio of 'best health' to 'worst health' areas		**9.1**	**2.8**	**6.5**	**1.3**	**0.9**
1	Glasgow Shettleston	92	7,970	289	95,148	25,822
2	Glasgow Springburn	63	7,214	132	105,946	29,646
3	Glasgow Maryhill	116	11,332	301	121,641	28,829
4	Glasgow Pollok	181	12,291	392	119,436	26,238
5	Glasgow Anniesland	224	13,629	931	121,297	27,465
6	Glasgow Baillieston	254	11,698	414	114,913	26,866
7	Manchester Central	345	15,970	1,749	185,785	38,032
8	Glasgow Govan	317	14,791	1,450	113,782	27,777
9	Liverpool Riverside	275	13,760	2,835	172,609	38,038
10	Manchester Blackley	336	18,677	1,476	174,383	36,199
11	Greenock and Inverclyde	363	15,512	1,302	110,733	25,490
12	Salford	371	17,148	2,313	159,407	34,249
13	Tyne Bridge	208	14,080	1,714	162,723	37,202
14	Glasgow Kelvin	199	13,656	1,185	102,117	27,741
15	Southwark North and Bermondsey	352	18,310	358	148,641	39,386
'Worst health' million		*3,696*	*206,038*	*16,841*	*2,008,561*	*468,980*
Rank	**Name**					
1	Wokingham	2,709	46,195	9,966	185,769	31,794
2	Woodspring	2,378	44,007	8,636	191,208	33,617
3	Romsey	2,617	42,963	8,013	180,463	31,702
4	Sheffield Hallam	1,246	30,612	7,500	161,759	28,782
5	South Cambridgeshire	2,474	43,744	9,008	195,260	33,590
6	Chesham and Amersham	3,546	47,895	10,280	197,802	33,237
7	South Norfolk	2,407	47,136	7,897	214,169	37,612
8	West Chelmsford	2,152	43,601	6,586	200,870	37,568
9	South Suffolk	2,227	39,743	7,139	182,638	32,669
10	Witney	2,602	45,668	6,816	197,169	35,412
11	Esher and Walton	3,261	50,783	10,371	219,150	38,063
12	Northavon	3,045	49,961	8,227	204,727	36,083
13	Buckingham	2,837	41,878	8,483	171,532	29,276
'Best health' million		*33,501*	*574,186*	*108,922*	*2,502,516*	*439,405*
Britain		873,053	20,528,433	2,860,101	110,498,578	21,619,998

Source: Analysis by authors of the 1991 Census of population

Figure 2.14: Total number of cars in the extreme areas of Britain (1991)

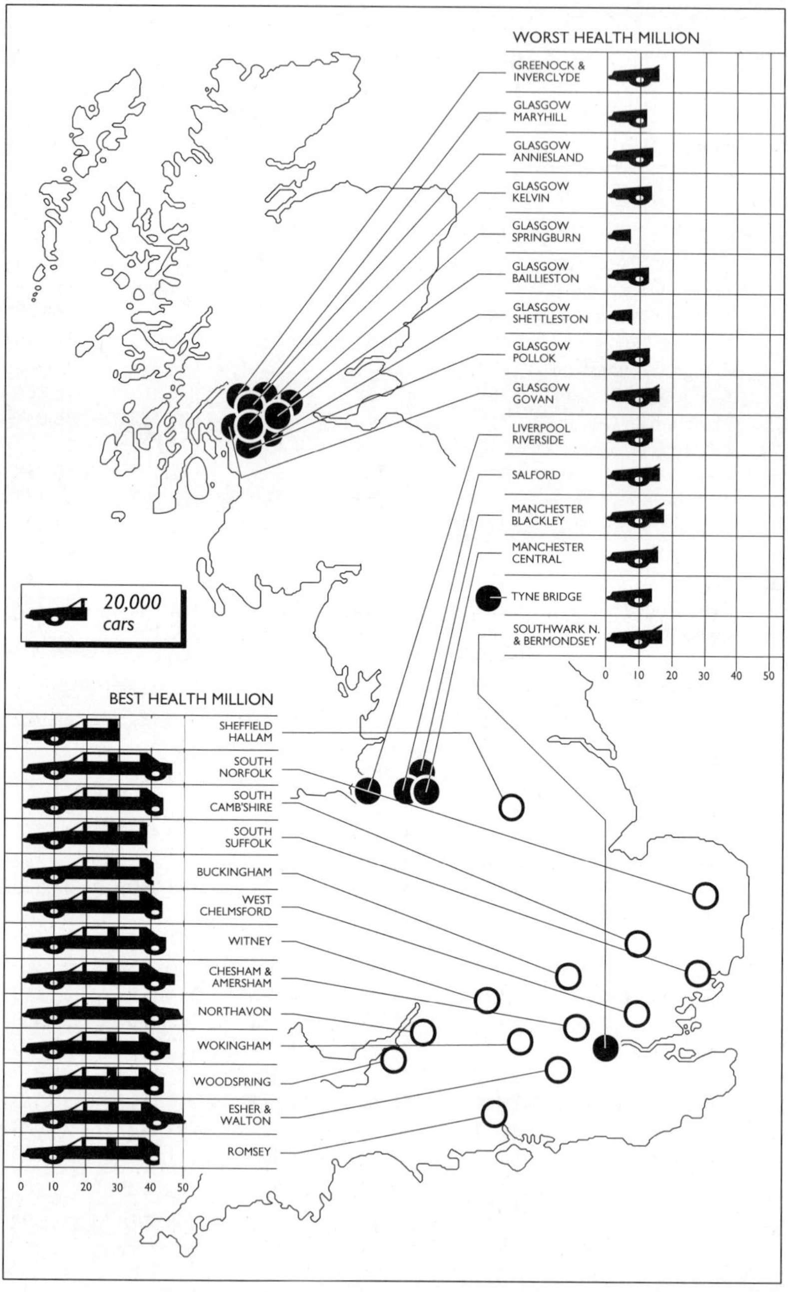

Source: Table 2.19

Retirement

The last phase of the life-course that we consider in this chapter is retirement. Although the health gap we have been concerned with throughout this chapter is mortality under age 65, the results of this gap have many influences upon people in retirement. Most directly, premature death (before the age of 65) leaves many more people widows or widowers in the 'worst health' areas of Britain compared to the 'best health' areas. As Table 2.20 shows, when aged 75-84 women in the 'worst health' areas are 60% less likely to be married than in the 'best health' areas. This difference is not due to differing rates of marriage, but to differing rates of widowhood. Figure 2.15 shows graphically how fewer women continue to be married in old age in the 'worst health' areas because men there are more likely to die relatively early in life. The difference between men and women is clear from Table 2.20.

Conclusion – poverty and health from the cradle to the grave

In this chapter we have shown how life chances in contemporary Britain vary. From infancy to old age, across the country and between different groups in society, life chances are unequal and become more unequal as people's lives progress. At the root of the differences observed are differences in the degrees of poverty experienced by different people, groups of people and in different areas.

We have seen that a mixture of factors result in our two groups of one million people having such differing chances in life and in death. The 'worst health' areas tend to also be the poorest areas and the 'best health' areas are much wealthier. Some of these factors are individual, but people's chances in life are also influenced by the community around them, whether this is through their chances at school, their chances in the job market, the availability of housing in their area or the prevailing rates of illness. Both geographically and temporally the influence of these factors is cumulative, as we have demonstrated in the maps and tables throughout this chapter. The 'worst health' areas also tend to be among those places with the fewest jobs available, with the poorest housing, the least cars and consequently some of the poorest children in Britain. The areas where the best health is found among the population also contain people who will find gaining employment most straightforward, where housing is of good quality and spacious, where there are more cars than there are families to use them and where very few children ever grow up in poverty.

Table 2.20: Marriage rate by age in the extreme areas of Britain (1991)

			Married people aged 65-74		Married people aged 75-84	
Rank	Name	Aged 65-84	Men %	Women %	Men %	Women %
	Ratio of 'worst health' to 'best health' areas	1.1	0.8	0.7	0.8	0.6
1	Glasgow Shettleston	9,716	60	35	48	16
2	Glasgow Springburn	9,953	60	38	50	18
3	Glasgow Maryhill	10,332	65	39	52	17
4	Glasgow Pollok	11,355	71	41	60	20
5	Glasgow Anniesland	13,253	71	45	60	21
6	Glasgow Baillieston	8,605	69	44	57	20
7	Manchester Central	12,693	55	40	47	18
8	Glasgow Govan	9,682	67	37	55	17
9	Liverpool Riverside	12,668	56	37	48	17
10	Manchester Blackley	13,725	65	45	57	22
11	Greenock and Inverclyde	9,955	69	43	61	19
12	Salford	12,664	61	42	51	19
13	Tyne Bridge	12,009	60	41	53	20
14	Glasgow Kelvin	9,113	59	36	53	17
15	Southwark North and Bermondsey	12,181	64	45	54	22
	'Worst health' million	167,904	63	41	54	19
Rank	**Name**					
1	Wokingham	7,624	84	57	70	27
2	Woodspring	12,656	84	60	73	32
3	Romsey	11,469	82	59	72	32
4	Sheffield Hallam	11,555	84	57	70	28
5	South Cambridgeshire	11,787	84	60	70	32
6	Chesham and Amersham	11,344	83	57	71	30
7	South Norfolk	15,860	82	61	71	34
8	West Chelmsford	11,941	83	57	70	30
9	South Suffolk	12,865	82	59	69	30
10	Witney	12,230	82	59	72	31
11	Esher and Walton	14,469	83	57	74	31
12	Northavon	10,346	83	59	71	31
13	Buckingham	9,107	82	58	70	32
	'Best health' million	153,253	83	59	71	31
Britain		7,976,805	77	53	66	27

Source: Analysis by authors of the 1991 Census of population

Figure 2.15: **Married women aged 75-84 in the extreme areas of Britain (1991)**

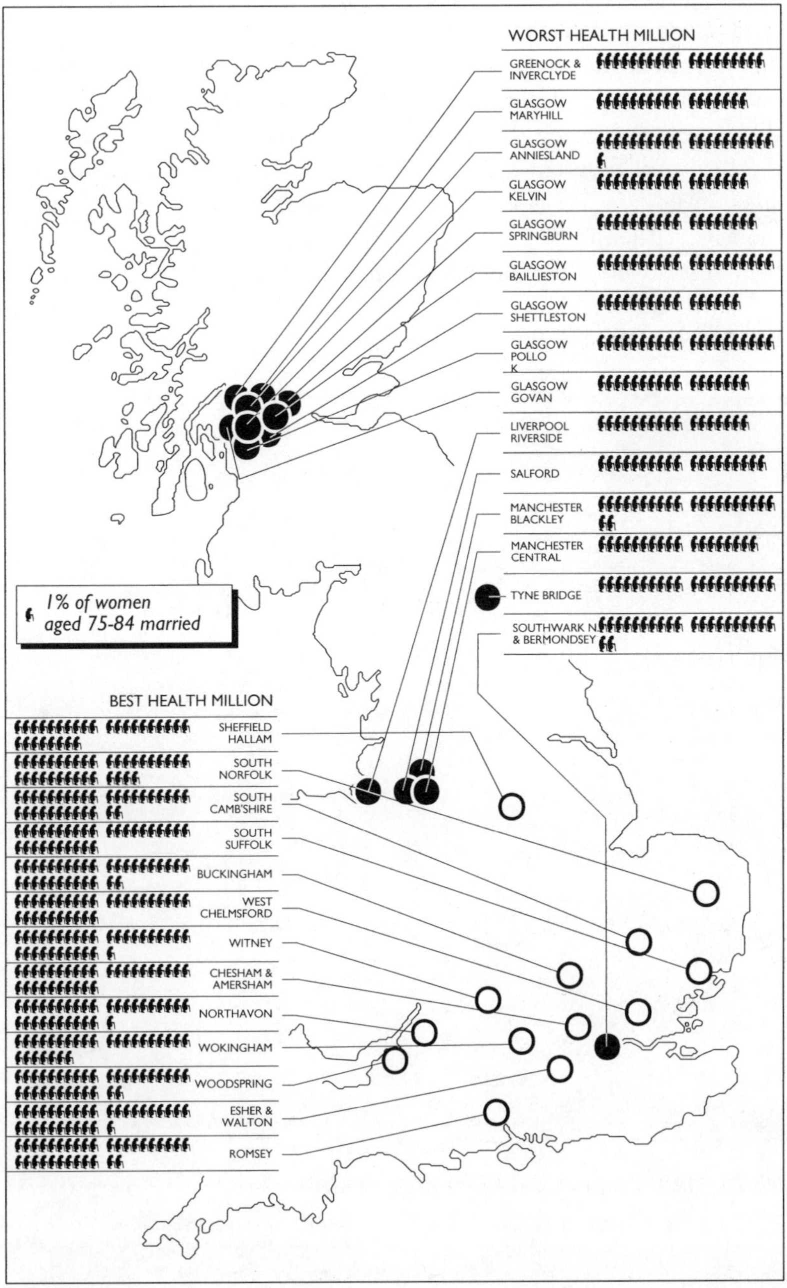

WORST HEALTH MILLION

GREENOCK & INVERCLYDE
GLASGOW MARYHILL
GLASGOW ANNIESLAND
GLASGOW KELVIN
GLASGOW SPRINGBURN
GLASGOW BAILLIESTON
GLASGOW SHETTLESTON
GLASGOW POLLOK
GLASGOW GOVAN
LIVERPOOL RIVERSIDE
SALFORD
MANCHESTER BLACKLEY
MANCHESTER CENTRAL
TYNE BRIDGE
SOUTHWARK N & BERMONDSEY

1% of women aged 75-84 married

BEST HEALTH MILLION

SHEFFIELD HALLAM
SOUTH NORFOLK
SOUTH CAMB'SHIRE
SOUTH SUFFOLK
BUCKINGHAM
WEST CHELMSFORD
WITNEY
CHESHAM & AMERSHAM
NORTHAVON
WOKINGHAM
WOODSPRING
ESHER & WALTON
ROMSEY

Source: Table 2.20

What is more, people migrate between these two groups of areas. Although very few go directly between the extreme areas, the effect of this migration is to conflate these differences. Over time, rich people tend to move into rich places and poor people into poor places, partly carrying their life chances with them, through the impact places have had on their lives up until migration (Brimblecombe et al, 1999). It is thus hardly surprising that we find such extreme differences between the health of different groups of people in Britain. The factors that affect health are also those which affect where you can choose to live – there is a self-reinforcing cycle of wealth accumulating wealth and poverty begetting poverty. This operates both across space – through migration – and over time – through the advantages rich children gain from growing up in rich areas and the disadvantages poor children suffer from living in poor areas.

THREE

Explaining the gap

Summary

- Social circumstances across the entire life-course – from birth through to late adulthood – influence people's health and well-being.

- The characteristics of the areas in which people live, as well as their individual characteristics, influence their health.

- Health differentials are primarily related to the lifetime material well-being of social groups, not to the psychological effects of position within hierarchies.

- Different socio-economic indicators – income, wealth, educational attainment and occupational group – are all related to and help explain people's health status.

- Educational attainment, as an indicator of socio-economic position, is primarily related to health through the advantages it gives people in their later socio-economic trajectories, not simply because education encourages healthy behaviours.

- Health inequalities are produced by the clustering of disadvantage – in opportunity, material circumstances and behaviours related to health – across people's lives.

- Health-related behaviours – such as smoking and diet – are strongly influenced by the social environment in which people live. People do not have equal choices about how they live their lives.

- Increasing inequalities in health over recent decades reflect the increasing polarisation of life chances – of opportunities, of material circumstances and of behaviours related to health.

- Reducing health inequalities requires that the underlying causes of these inequalities are tackled.

Introduction

Chapter 2 demonstrated the existence of large inequalities in health within Britain and Chapter 4 will show that these inequalities are increasing. This is true for both sexes, for different age groups and for morbidity as well as mortality. Chapter 5 will also show that there are inequalities in the provision and uptake of some medical services. There are large and often increasing inequalities in the many factors which could underlie observed health differentials, ranging from income, threat of unemployment and unfavourable characteristics of residential areas, through to cigarette smoking. However, simply demonstrating that there are strong associations does not prove causal links. In this chapter, a more analytical approach is used to investigate (to the extent that this is currently possible) the causes of inequalities in health.

One way to begin to understand which aspects of the social environment produce inequalities in health is to explore which indicators of socio-economic position are the key measures which differentiate between people at different levels of risk of ill-health and death. Socio-economic circumstances across the entire life-course – from infancy to old age – are of importance. Much of the evidence for this is ecological, that is, at the area or group level, rather than the individual level. For instance, we know that areas where children are likely to live in poverty also tend to have high infant and child mortality rates.

Ecological associations cannot be automatically extrapolated to individuals (for example, not all people living in rich areas are rich), therefore it is important to note that a great deal of research using follow-up studies of individuals has shown that the cumulative effect of favourable or unfavourable social experiences determines health status. Such studies – called 'cohort studies' – take a sample of individuals and follow them over a number of years to see which factors are associated with subsequent ill-health and early death. A broad view of the possible causes of health inequalities must be taken, one which encapsulates not just what is happening to people at a particular time, but what has happened to them in the past and even before they were born. The high infant mortality rates of babies born in Glasgow today, for example, can be traced back to the poverty which became increasingly concentrated in these areas during the industrial decline which began 30 years ago.

In this chapter we argue that when the importance of socio-economic circumstances across the whole life-course is considered it shows how inadequate singular explanations of inequalities in health are. Singular explanations in terms of particular health-related behaviours or stress processes do little to explain the extent of health inequalities seen today. The demonstration of the importance of the wider ecological contexts of people's lives takes us even further away from singular explanations. If health inequalities can be shown to arise primarily from inequalities in socio-economic circumstances, which in turn arise from the differences in opportunities between communities and classes of people, then it is these divides which have to be redressed if health inequalities are to be reduced.

After examining lifetime social circumstances, it is necessary to look at indicators of socio-economic position which have been used in health statistics, such as education, occupation, income, the characteristics of residential areas and access to assets such as a car or a home which is owned rather than rented. If it is found that any one dimension of social position is of particular importance then, clearly, explanations for inequalities in health would have to focus on this dimension of social experience. One approach to this question is to see whether adverse social circumstances at different stages of the life-course have particular effects on different causes of ill-health. If this is found to be the case, then the focus of the search for factors underlying the social distribution of a particular cause of ill-health should turn to the relevant life-course stage.

Lifetime social circumstances

In the previous chapter it was seen that infant mortality (the death of infants before they reach their first birthday) and the health status of children are strongly related to the social circumstances of their parents and the wider communities in which they live. The social environment for infants and children will be largely determined by parental circumstances and how these change. Once children become adults there is a longer period over which social circumstances might change. Transition from the parental home to more independent living arrangements, transition from education into employment or non-employment and changes in family circumstances and employment situation through the working years and beyond will all be important. However, the 'inequalities in health' literature has tended to treat social circumstances as a static phenomenon, analysing the health of adults by their current (or main) occupation, for example. More recently, the importance of social circumstances throughout life has been recognised

(Mare, 1990; Ben–Shlomo and Davey Smith, 1991; Davey Smith et al, 1994, 1997; Wunsch et al, 1996), as the following examples illustrate.

The 1958 birth cohort

The influence of lifetime social circumstances with respect to morbidity has been well illustrated using data from the 1958 birth cohort. This study involved all children born in England, Wales and Scotland during one week in 1958. Follow–up surveys were conducted when the cohort members were aged 7, 11, 16, 23 and 33 years, with over 10,000 study participants being included at each phase. This large, representative study provides data for a detailed examination of the development of inequalities in health throughout childhood and into the adulthood years (Power et al, 1991, 1996, 1997, 1998, 1999; Power and Matthews, 1997). Self-rated poor health at age 33 showed large social class gradients (Table 3.1) whether social class at birth (ie based on parental occupation) or social class of cohort members in 1991 at age 33 was used (Power et al, 1997). There is a clear and striking trend of increasing risk of being in poor health moving from social classes I and II to IV and V, with more than twice the risk of being in poor health in the latter than the former classes. Social class at birth will be an indicator for social circumstances in early childhood, while social class at age 33 will be an indicator of circumstances in adulthood. Social class at birth and in adulthood are related but, within this study, analyses demonstrate that both make independent contributions to inequalities in poor health in adulthood (Power et al, 1999). A lifetime social position score was based on occupational social class of fathers at each cohort member's birth and at age 16, and each cohort member's own social class at 23 and 33. This score ranged from 4 to 16 and demonstrated a very strong association with the experience of poor health at age 33 (see Figure 3.1). Greater than fivefold differences in prevalence of poor health at 33 are seen (Power et al, 1999).

Table 3.1: 1958 birth cohort prevalence of poor health* at age 33 by social class at different stages of the life-course (% of population reporting poor health in each social class group), Britain (1958-91)

| Social class | Men | | Women | |
	Social class at birth	Social class at 33	Social class at birth	Social class at 33
I & II	7.9	8.5	7.2	9.4
IIINM	10.2	13.3	9.2	11.4
IIIM	12.7	14.4	14.5	15.5
IV & V	16.4	17.7	17.6	18.8
Ratio IV&V:I&II	**2.1**	**2.1**	**2.4**	**2.0**

Note: * Participants who consider their health to be 'fair' or 'poor'.
Source: Power et al (1996, 1997)

Figure 3.1: **Poor health at age 33 and cumulative socio-economic circumstances (birth to age 33), Britain (1958-91)**

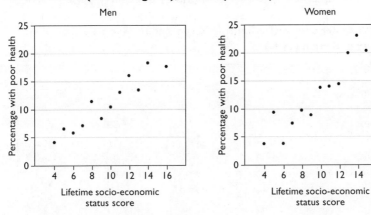

Note: 'Poor health' includes subjects who rated their health as 'fair'.
Source: Power et al (1999)

The Breadline Britain *survey and other surveys of poverty*

Representative surveys that are specifically designed to measure poverty, such as the *Breadline Britain* survey (conducted in 1983 and 1990) referred to in Chapter 2, have provided considerable evidence on the substantial health gap between poor people and the rest of society (as we saw in Figures 2.3 and 2.10). For example, the 1985/86 Booth Centenary Poverty Survey of London (Townsend et al, 1987) found that people living in poverty were almost ten times more likely to consider themselves as having poor health; respondents were twice as likely to report having had an illness in the previous two weeks and more than three times as likely to report having had a major health problem in the last year, than were the rest of Londoners. Similarly, the 1990 *Breadline Britain* survey found that poor people were 1.6 times more likely to suffer from a long-standing illness, 5.4 times more likely to suffer from feeling isolated and 5.5 times more likely to feel depressed (Pantazis and Gordon, 1997). Furthermore, the health gap was found to be even larger if survey respondents' intensity and history of poverty was taken into account. Figure 3.2 illustrates that there is a clear linear relationship between long-standing illness and a person's history of poverty.

Figure 3.2: Per cent with a limiting long-standing illness by history of poverty in Britain (1990)

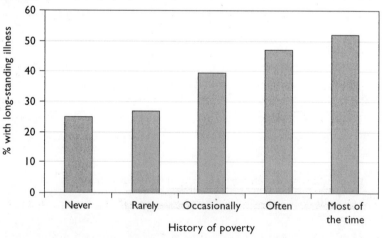

Note: Question 16 of the *Breadline Britain* survey asked: 'Do you think you could genuinely say you are poor now, all the time, sometimes, or never?' Respondents thus may interpret 'now' as either today, the past week, past month or occasionally during the past year, depending on their usual budgeting period and the frequency of receiving income.
Source: Analysis by authors of the *Breadline Britain* survey

Figure 3.3: **Per cent feeling isolated and depressed by present level of poverty, Britain (1990)**

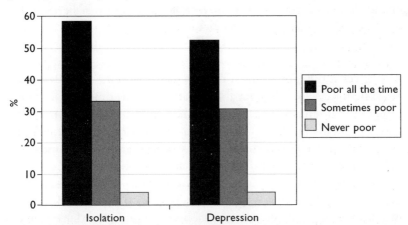

Note: Question 17 of the *Breadline Britain* survey asked: 'Looking back over your adult life, how often have there been times in your life when you think you have lived in poverty by the standards of that time?' This will be interpreted by most people as their whole adult life, and so the time period of reference will vary by age.

Source: Analysis by authors of the *Breadline Britain* survey

Similarly, Figure 3.3 illustrates that there is a clear relationship between a respondent's intensity of poverty and his or her feeling of isolation and depression. People who were 'poor all the time' were more than ten times more likely to feel isolated and depressed than people who were 'never poor' (Payne, 1997).

The *Breadline Britain* surveys demonstrate a clear dose/response relationship between poverty and poor physical and mental health at the individual level. The worse the poverty and deprivation experienced by a person and the longer these conditions persist, the worse the person's health is likely to be.

The Collaborative Study

The 1958 birth cohort, referred to above, allows us to understand the socio-economic influences on the development of morbidity during childhood and early adulthood. The risk of dying is also influenced by the cumulative effect of social circumstances across life. In a study of nearly 6,000 men aged 35-64 in the West of Scotland who were followed up for 20 years (Davey Smith et al, 1997), the risk of death was related to the occupational social class of their fathers (an indicator of their social circumstances in early life), the occupational social class of their first job on entering the labour market and their occupational social class at the time they entered the study. Men with fathers from a manual social class had a more than 40% higher risk of death than men with non-manual social class fathers. Men who were in manual social class occupations themselves at the time of the study also had around 40% higher risk of death than men in non-manual occupations at this time. Men whose first job was in a manual occupation had around a third higher mortality risk than men whose first job was non-manual. An index of lifetime social circumstances was constructed by simply adding the number of occasions at which each participant's class location was manual or non-manual. This could range from '3 manual' – for the men whose fathers had manual occupations, whose first occupation at labour market entry was manual and who were in manual occupations at the time of entry into the study – to '3 non-manual', for men whose fathers were in non-manual occupations, whose first job at labour market entry was non-manual and who were in non-manual occupations at the time of entry into the study. Figure 3.4 presents death rates from all-causes and from cardiovascular disease according to this cumulative social class measure.

Figure 3.4: Age-adjusted death rates (per 10,000 years) over 21 years of follow-up for men according to cumulative social class, the Collaborative Study, West of Scotland (1970-94)

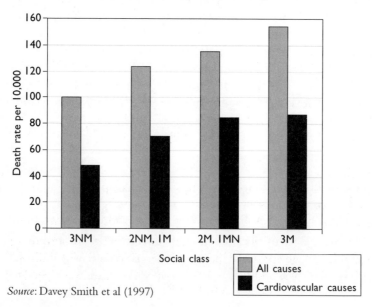

Source: Davey Smith et al (1997)

To reiterate, the risk of dying in later adulthood is influenced by social circumstances acting in childhood and then throughout adult life. The focus of most investigations of inequalities in health has been on adulthood social circumstances, which has meant that the contribution of lifetime socio-economic conditions to mortality risk has been little investigated. However, other studies from Britain, the US and Norway have similarly demonstrated the cumulative influence of lifetime social experience on adulthood morbidity and mortality risk (Mare, 1990; Salhi et al, 1995; Wunsch et al, 1996; Wannamethee et al, 1996). The independent influences of social circumstances in childhood and in later life on ill-health and the risk of dying in adulthood indicate that a search for the causes of inequalities in health must be a broad-based one and must include all stages of the life-course.

Dimensions of socio-economic position

The Longitudinal Study

As discussed in the preceding chapter, several dimensions of socio-economic position can be distinguished. These include occupation, education, income, assets, wealth and other characteristics of residential area. With respect to overall health measures – such as all-cause death rates, subjective ratings of general health or the prevalence of a long-standing illness – these different dimensions demonstrate the same general associations with health outcomes. In Figures 3.5 and 3.6 data from the Longitudinal Study (LS) (the follow-up of people from the 1971 Census) are used to relate mortality to several socio-economic indicators simultaneously (Goldblatt, 1990b). The different dimensions of socio-economic position tend to all contribute to the prediction of health outcomes. This is illustrated further in the tables below. For example, within occupational social classes, indicators of material well-being – such as car ownership and housing tenure – are associated with lower death rates (Table 3.2 and Figure 3.7). Cars themselves are unlikely to increase people's life expectancy (indeed driving a car can be dangerous), but as an indicator of available income and hence of favourable socio-economic circumstances they are a sensitive measure. Occasionally car driving can, of course, be safer than walking, as is thought to be the case where children are safer as passengers inside cars than they are when crossing the road in front of them. This is thought to be one of the explanations for the socio-economic inequalities found between children's life chances discussed in Chapter 2.

Figure 3.5: **SMRs of men aged 15-64 by educational level and social class, England and Wales (1976-81)**

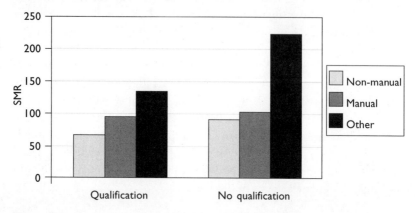

Note: 'Other' includes men who could not be assigned a class because they had no work in 1971.
Source: Goldblatt (1990b)

Figure 3.6: **SMRs of married women aged 15-64 by own and husband's social class, England and Wales (1976-81)**

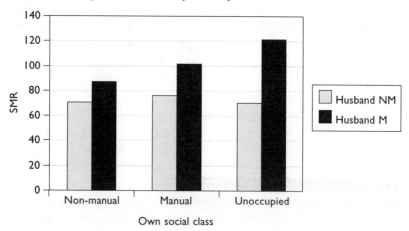

Note: 'Unoccupied' includes people who could not be assigned a class because they had no work in 1971.
Source: Goldblatt (1990b)

Table 3.2: **SMRs for men aged 15-59 by housing tenure and car access, England and Wales (1976-91)**

	Car access			No car access			All households
	Owner-occupied	Privately rented	Local authority	Owner-occupied	Privately rented	Local authority	
I & II	67	80	93	92	120	130	75
IV & V	98	101	105	113	124	125	114
All classes	78	93	106	108	128	129	100

Note: These SMRs are slightly different from those presented in Table 2.18, which also draws on the LS, as the time period and age groups being studied are different. However, the overall pattern is the same.
Source: Goldblatt (1990b)

Thus whether we use educational qualifications (Figure 3.5), occupational social class (Figure 3.6), housing tenure or car access (Table 3.2 and Figure 3.7) we find that those who are more advantaged have better relative life chances. In Chapter 2 we showed how these factors were coincident geographically; here we are demonstrating how they are cumulative socially.

Figure 3.7: **SMRs of women aged 15-59 by housing tenure and car access, England and Wales (1976-81)**

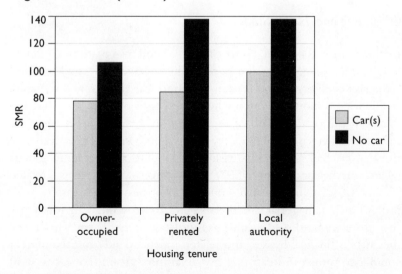

Source: Goldblatt (1990b)

The Whitehall study

In the Whitehall study a large group of male civil servants from London have been followed up since the early 1970s. Employment grade within the civil service is a powerful indicator of death rates. Furthermore, car ownership predicts mortality risk within each employment grade. Two decades ago the greatest differential within middle-aged men in the non-manual groups, that between social class III non-manual and social class I, was only 30% (OPCS, 1978). However once civil servants' employment grade and car access are taken into account differences of over 300% are found between different groups of non-manual workers (Davey Smith et al, 1990a). Clerical staff without cars had a mortality rate over three times that of car-owning administrators. Both administrators and clerical workers fall into the non-manual social class groups. This demonstrates that the use of more precise indicators of socio-economic position can lead to finer discrimination of the material well-being of groups, which in turn leads to greater mortality differentials being observed. The use of multiple indicators provides a proxy for levels of poverty, income and wealth (in other words material well-being) among the population. Someone who is poor is likely to own neither a home nor a car. As income and wealth increase, so do assets, hence the ownership of assets is strongly associated with health through the levels of available income and wealth – and well-being – that this implies.

British Regional Heart Study

In the British Regional Heart Study – a follow-up study of nearly 8,000 middle-aged men from 24 towns in England, Wales and Scotland – the risk of dying was associated with both car and home ownership. As Figure 3.8 shows, the men who owned both of these assets had less than half the risk of death of the men who owned neither (here we refer to relative risks, see Glossary). The men owning one or other of these assets had a mortality risk between the two extreme groups (Wannamethee and Shaper, 1997). Occupational social class was related to the risk of dying within groups who possessed these assets, with professional/managerial (social class I and II) groups having lower risk than the semi/unskilled manual groups (social class IV and V). Several measures of ill-health were also related independently to the different socio-economic indicators. For example, around one tenth of professional/managerial men who owned both a car and a home reported not being in good health, while over half of semi/unskilled manual men who owned neither a car nor a home reported this.

Figure 3.8: **Car and home ownership and adjusted* relative risk (RR) of mortality for all-causes, cardiovascular disease, cancer and other causes – men, Britain (1978-92)**

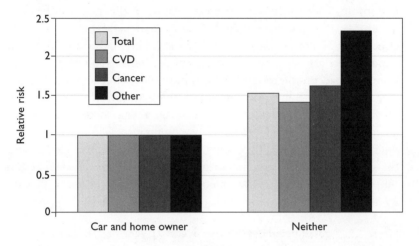

Note: *Adjusted for age, smoking, body mass index (BMI), physical activity, alcohol intake, height, cholesterol, systolic blood pressure and social class.
Source: Wannamethee and Shaper (1997)

Within this general pattern, the British Regional Heart Study investigators noted that for men who were neither car nor homeowners, occupational social class had little influence on mortality. They interpreted this as demonstrating that material well-being is the major factor determining the differences in mortality observed between social groups. This interpretation argues against occupational social class differences being somehow due to social status – that is, to the psychological effects of standing within a social hierarchy – since higher social classes will be of higher status whether or not they own or can afford assets such as a car or home. This apparent primacy of material well-being will be returned to later.

Education and health

In the US and some European countries, education has been a widely used socio-economic indicator, probably because information regarding education is the main socio-economic measure contained in national data sets (Krieger and Fee, 1994). Similarly, occupational social class and asset ownership have been used in Britain because actual measures of material well-being are difficult to collect. While the decision to use education as the primary socio-economic indicator in these circumstances may be largely influenced by data availability, the choice of indicator can influence the interpretation of the observed socio-economic health differentials. For example, the health effects of occupational hazards in unskilled manual jobs depend directly on work conditions, and reducing socio-economic differentials caused by such exposures requires changing work environments. Conversely, health differences according to level of education have been attributed to the direct effects of education, including the acquisition of knowledge regarding health-damaging behaviours, the ability to optimise use of health services, the development of time preferences favourable to health maintenance, an increasing willingness to invest in human capital, and the promotion of the psychological attributes of high self-esteem and self-efficacy (Fuchs, 1979; Winkleby et al, 1992; Pincus and Callahan, 1994).

Figure 3.9: **Age-adjusted death rates over a 21-year period for men according to social class (per 10,000 person years), the Collaborative Study, West of Scotland (1970-94)**

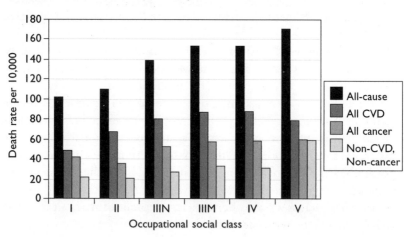

Source: Davey Smith et al (1998b)

Figure 3.10: Age-adjusted death rates (per 10,000 years) over 21 years of follow-up for men according to age at leaving full-time education, the Collaborative Study, West of Scotland (1970-94)

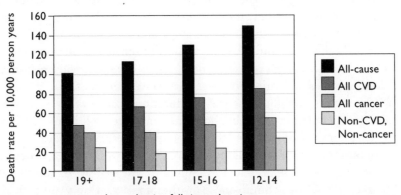

Source: Davey Smith et al (1998b)

In the West of Scotland Collaborative Study mentioned above, the risk of dying was strongly associated with both social class in adulthood and with an index of educational attainment: the age of leaving full-time education (Figures 3.9 and 3.10). However what is not shown in the figures is that when taking both indicators of socio-economic position into account (Davey Smith et al, 1998b), the graded association between social class and overall mortality appeared within each education category while, within social class groups, the relationship between education and mortality was less clear. This suggests that lifetime social circumstances, rather than the psychosocial effects of education, are the key determinants of health inequalities. Similarly, cigarette smoking was more strongly related to occupational social class than education (see 'Education and smoking' below). This suggests that it is the social environment in adulthood that initiates, or maintains, smoking behaviour. Education is, of course, related to smoking behaviour, but this appears to be mainly through its influence on occupation in adulthood.

As seen in Chapter 2, the differences in educational attainment at age 15 between the 'worst health' and 'best health' areas of Britain are relatively small (at least when compared to the differences in mortality rates). This is partly a result of the British state education system which, since the introduction of comprehensive education, has reduced inequalities between children (by not 'failing' the majority at age 11, although inequalities in tertiary education are increasing, see Figure 4.15).

However, it provides further (albeit ecological) evidence that inequalities in education are not the key determinants of health inequalities – inequalities in material well-being throughout life are the key.

At the individual level, when different causes of death were examined in the Collaborative Study, the only group of causes which demonstrated a strong association with education, after adulthood occupational social class had been taken into account, was death from cardiovascular disease. This is consistent with education being an indicator of socio-economic circumstances in childhood and factors related to this. Parents' circumstances strongly influence the educational career of their children and thus people in worse childhood circumstances will be more likely to have finished full-time education at an earlier age. Adverse socio-economic conditions in childhood have been shown to be of particular importance with respect to cardiovascular disease risk in adulthood (Barker, 1994; Davey Smith and Ben-Shlomo, 1997; Davey Smith et al, 1997, 1998c; Wannamethee and Shaper, 1997).

Education and ill-health

In the 1958 birth cohort (discussed earlier in this chapter) level of education and lifetime social class were related to prevalence of poor health at age 33. Both were associated with poor health, and as in the Collaborative Study when they were considered together social class was the more important indicator of health status (Power et al, 1999).

Education and smoking

The main conclusion from the findings regarding education and occupational social class is that both are strongly related to ill-health and mortality, but that there is no evidence that education plays a predominant role in this regard. In fact the reverse appears to be the case. These data suggest that both education and social class are serving as indices of life-course socio-economic experience and material well-being. In this sense, education is important because of the opportunities it creates for improving material conditions of life which follow the completion of formal education, rather than for any specific effects of education itself. Thus, in the Collaborative Study smoking behaviour was more strongly related to occupational social class than to education. If education had its influence through the ability to assimilate health-related knowledge, then the reverse would have been expected, since even when the Collaborative Study was started in the early 1970s there was already a considerable amount of publicity regarding the health-damaging effects of cigarette smoking. This is consistent with studies which show that education remains related to smoking even after health-related knowledge has been taken into account (Kenkel, 1991). The influence of education on smoking relates to the better social environment that education buys for people in adulthood, rather than simply through giving people access to knowledge.

Education and mental health

Occupational social class and education have also been investigated in relation to neurotic disorder in a representative sample of over 10,000 people in the UK (Lewis et al, 1998). Each participant was interviewed and psychological problems – neurotic disorder (mainly depression and anxiety) – identified. Neurotic disorder was associated with housing tenure (around double the prevalence in people renting compared to those who owned their homes), car access – with a gradient of decreasing risk from no car, to one car, to two cars – occupational social class and educational qualifications (Tables 3.3, 3.4 and 3.5).

Table 3.3: **Odds ratios for neurotic disorder by sex, housing tenure and car access, UK (1993)**

	Men	**Women**
Housing tenure		
Owner	1.0	1.0
Renter	2.17	1.71
Car access		
Two or more	1.0	1.0
One car	1.45	1.49
No car	2.59	2.25

Note: Adjusted for age and household size.
Source: Lewis et al (1998)

Table 3.4: **Odds ratios for neurotic disorder by sex and social class, UK (1993)**

Social class	Men	Women
I	1.0	1.0
II	2.47	0.95
IIIN	2.84	1.14
IIIM	2.41	1.32
IV	2.20	1.52
V	2.74	1.43

Note: Adjusted for age and household size.
Source: Lewis et al (1998)

Table 3.5: **Odds ratios for neurotic disorder by sex and educational qualifications, UK (1993)**

Educational qualifications	Men	Women
'A' level or above	1.0	1.0
GCSE grades A-C or equivalent	1.27	0.98
GCSE grades D-F or equivalent	1.14	1.21
No qualifications	1.29	1.26

Note: Adjusted for age and household size.
Source: Lewis et al (1998)

The direct indicators of material well-being – home ownership and car access – demonstrated the strongest association with neurotic disorder and were the indicators which remained associated with neurotic disorder when all of the indicators were analysed simultaneously. Neurotic disorder, therefore, seems to be most strongly associated with a low standard of living, rather than with specific aspects of education or with the component of occupational social class related to position in a hierarchy (and the possible psychological consequences of this). As is the case with mortality (Wannamethee and Shaper, 1997), the different levels of material well-being experienced by different occupational groups seems to be key.

Communities and socio-economic position

The population characteristics of areas of residence are increasingly being used as indicators of socio-economic position; indeed this was our approach throughout the preceding chapter. For example, Census data can be used to categorise places as deprived (with a low proportion of owner-occupiers, a high proportion of households without access to a car, a high proportion of residents who are semi-skilled or unskilled manual workers, a high unemployment rate and a high proportion of overcrowded homes, for example) or affluent, at the other end of the spectrum. Such area-based measures can be considered in two different ways. First, they can be viewed as proxy markers for the socio-economic position of individuals. Often it is difficult to obtain individual-level data but it is possible to know where people live and thus assign a deprivation score to them. When conceptualised in this way, area-based measures would be considered to be rather crude measures of socio-economic position, since they will misclassify some individuals, for example, wealthy people living in deprived areas or poor people living in more affluent areas. Area-based measures may, however, not simply serve as indicators of the socio-economic position of individuals. There is a second way they can be interpreted, as indicators of an additional – and non-individual – aspect of socio-economic position. Areas with a high level of socio-economic disadvantage may also be disadvantaged with respect to transport, retail outlets, leisure facilities, environmental pollution, and social disorganisation, in ways that influence health independently of the socio-economic characteristics of the people living in these areas (Macintyre et al, 1993). The demonstration of area-based effects would be important in emphasising the need to focus health promotion initiatives on the broader characteristics of places where disadvantaged people live, rather than simply on the people who live in these areas.

The areas in which people live also have other broader implications for their lives. People are often stereotyped by their area of residence and this can have many direct effects on their lives and material well-being. Employers may be unwilling to employ people from certain parts of the city; the police and teachers may treat children from different housing estates differently. More directly, different areas are served by different schools, attendance at which gives children different chances of success at education and thereafter in employment. Different areas are served by different industries which pay people at different rates and which are more or less susceptible to closure and hence redundancies. Different areas have very different housing market values and hence most people cannot afford to live in the richest areas of Britain. People are excluded from these areas according to their levels of material well-being, while other areas only cater for people (through the state housing allocation system) who are poor enough to qualify to live there. This means that areas provide a good indicator of longer-term socio-economic position as 'permission' to live in particular areas depends on your (or your parents') levels of income and wealth in the past.

Area effects on individuals

The contribution of area-based and individual socio-economic indicators has been investigated in several studies (see for example, Congdon, 1995; Jones and Duncan, 1995; Shouls et al, 1998; Wiggins et al, 1998). Here we present evidence from a study of 15,000 men and women from the towns of Renfrew and Paisley in the West of Scotland (Davey Smith et al, 1998d). Both the area-based deprivation score and individually assigned occupational social class were strongly related to the risk of death (Table 3.6), with an independent association between each indicator and mortality. A wide range of characteristics of areas that are not simply reducible to the socio-economic characteristics of the people living in these areas but which reflect the broader social context have been related to mortality. These include such factors as socio-economic inequality within the areas, voting patterns at elections, crime rates, education services and medical care expenditure and welfare services (Kaplan et al, 1996; Ben-Shlomo et al, 1996; Kennedy et al, 1996; Davey Smith and Dorling, 1996).

Table 3.6: Relative rates of mortality by deprivation category, West of Scotland (1972-91)

	Deprivation category		
	1-3 (affluent)	4-5	6-7 (deprived)
Men			
All-cause mortality			
Age	1	1.27	1.47
Age + social class	1	1.19	1.34
Cardiovascular mortality			
Age	1	1.24	1.33
Age + social class	1	1.19	1.26
Women			
All-cause mortality			
Age	1	1.18	1.40
Age + social class	1	1.12	1.29
Cardiovascular mortality			
Age	1	1.28	1.48
Age + social class	1	1.18	1.33

Note: Relative rates are adjusted for age, and for age and social class. With the latter adjustment the influence of area-based deprivation on death after taking into account social class make up of affluent and deprived areas is seen.
Source: Davey Smith et al (1998d)

Most studies to date have tended to use socio–economic indicators that have essentially the same meaning at the individual level and when aggregated at the area level. Studies of particular areas have found that poorer areas contained people who were less likely to consume (and had less access to) healthy foods, less likely to participate in sport, more likely to be smokers, to be shorter, have higher body mass indices and greater waist–hip ratios (Ellaway and Macintyre, 1996; Ellaway et al, 1997). Factors which would allow for a healthier life – such as sports facilities, transport facilities, access to shops which sell healthy food at reasonable prices, absence of a threat of crime, etc – are more prevalent and more easily accessible in the more affluent areas. Many aspects of the physical and social environment of areas can affect health in a variety of ways, and therefore influence a range of health problems.

Importantly, within the particularly segregated society of Britain, different areas serve to collect people who have different chances in life as reflected by their ability to pay to move into and live in those areas. Furthermore, from living in these areas people's life chances are shaped in the future, most obviously through their ability to find employment in their area. It is thus hardly surprising that some of the greatest differences in health are found between the extreme areas of Britain identified in Chapter 2. It is, however, important to remember that these differences are the result of the playing out of over one million lives in each set of areas. There is a multitude of influences on those lives that results in death rates under age 65 being almost three times greater in one population than the other. These influences result partly from the effects on socio-economic position and material well-being of living in these areas (which in turn influence the distribution of facilities outlined above) but also from the histories of the people living in these places and these people's individual and family life histories which, in turn, shape and are shaped by the communities in which they live (Brimblecombe et al, 1999).

The role of migration

Many people will have moved into and out of these areas over the course of their lifetimes. The possible role of migration in explaining geographical patterns in mortality has been largely ignored. However, in a recent analysis we investigated this possibility (Davey Smith et al, 1998e). We found that areas with high mortality were also areas with high rates of population decline (see Figure 3.11).

Figure 3.11: Population change (aged under 65) between 1971 and 1991 and absolute change in SMR for deaths under 65 for British constituencies (1991-95 to 1981-85)

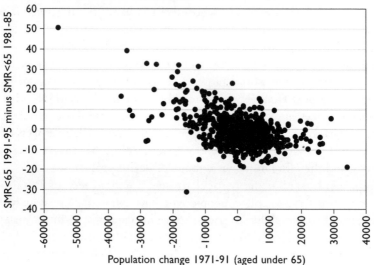

Population change 1971-91 (aged under 65)

Source: Analysis by authors

Figure 3.11 shows how the change in mortality ratio seen between 1981-85 and 1991-95 is related to the change in total population seen in the same areas 10 years earlier (the change in population between 1971 and 1991) for the 641 parliamentary constituencies we have been following. Five of the constituencies with the highest mortality rates in the early 1990s experienced the largest declines in population some 20 years earlier. These were: Glasgow Shettleston, Liverpool Riverside, Glasgow Springburn, Salford and Manchester Central, which lost between 56,000 and 32,000 mainly young people each, mostly due to out-migration in the 1970s. The people they left behind were consequently some of the most deprived in Britain. All the 'worst health' 15 constituencies lost at least 10,000 people aged under 65 in net terms between 1971 and 1981. The population loss was greatest in Glasgow Shettleston where the population aged under 65 fell from 108,000 in 1971 to 50,700 by 1991, a fall of over 50% within that geographical area. Only a small fraction of this decline was due to the high mortality rates in these areas. The main reason for these declines was massive net out-migration.

The fact that population change since the 1970s is so clearly related to mortality change in the 1980s suggests that people in Britain recognise

Artefact

At the time the Black Committee were reviewing the evidence on health inequalities there were several concerns regarding the quality of data which allowed for the description of these inequalities within Britain. For example, the main source of data on differences in death rates came from the Registrar General's Decennial Supplements which reported mortality rates for the different social classes around each Census. These mortality rates were constructed by relating death certificates – on which the main occupation of the deceased was recorded – to the number of people of that age group in the population at the time of the Census. This means that the source of information on occupation (and therefore on occupational social class) was different for the numerator – the deaths – than for the denominator – the number of people in each occupation (and thus social class) at the Census. Since there are different sources for these data – for example a surviving spouse or other relative in the case of some deaths, as opposed to the person themselves at the Census – bias may be introduced. The coding of social class from occupation can be an imprecise activity. Thus someone known as an 'engineer' could be a shop-floor worker (in the skilled manual, social class IIIM group) or a professional engineer in social class I (generally a non-shop-floor worker with a degree). The way someone's occupation is described could, then, lead them to being assigned either to social class IIIM or I. This could clearly lead to bias (known as numerator-denominator bias) in the mortality rates that are calculated.

Such issues generated considerable discussion, and eliminating bias of this kind was one reason why the Longitudinal Study – which we have discussed and from which we have presented data in this and the previous chapter – was set up. By linking deaths directly to information provided at the Census the possibility of numerator-denominator bias was eliminated. The Longitudinal Study, as we have shown earlier, yielded similar findings with respect to social class differences in mortality as had the Decennial Supplements. There was, therefore, little evidence that health inequalities were influenced by artefacts of this type. Several other categories of artefactual explanation for health inequalities have been advanced, but a detailed review of evidence on these suggests that they do not contribute in any substantial fashion to the generation of observed health differentials (Davey Smith et al, 1994). Indeed, the evidence suggests that far from artefacts producing or exaggerating the magnitude of health inequalities, data problems lead to existing inequalities being underestimated by conventional analyses. For example, as we have discussed earlier in this chapter, use of the Registrar General's occupational social class leads to the demonstration of considerably smaller inequalities in mortality than does the use of more precise measures of material circumstances. An overall assessment of the role of artefacts in explaining inequalities in health would be that they lead to artefactual attenuation – rather than exaggeration – of the magnitude and importance of these health differentials (Bloor et al, 1987; Davey Smith et al, 1994).

Social selection

At their crudest, artefact explanations of health inequalities suggest that the apparent differentials in health status between social groups are created by the processes of measurement and data analysis, rather than existing in their own right. Social selection explanations, conversely, accept that health and social position are linked, but suggest that the direction of causation is from health to social position rather than vice versa. Such interpretations are not novel – Edwin Chadwick, author of the famous *Report on the sanitary condition of the labouring population of Great Britain* originally published in 1842 sometimes suggested that the poor were living in straightened circumstances because sickness lead to an inability to earn a living, rather than because poverty generated ill-health.

The most straightforward selection argument is predicated on the notion that sick individuals move down the social hierarchy, and healthy individuals move up, leading to a concentration of people with a high risk of mortality at the lower end of the social spectrum, and a concentration of low-risk individuals at the upper extreme. If this process is considered to occur during the working life of individuals then it is referred to as intragenerational selection. Studies of this suggest that it is, at most, a very minor contributor to socio-economic differentials in health and mortality risk in adulthood (Blane et al, 1993). For example in the West of Scotland Collaborative Study, discussed earlier in this chapter, the group of men who started their working life in non-manual jobs and by middle age were in manual jobs – those people seen as having been downwardly mobile – had no worse health profiles than was to be expected on the basis of their lifetime social circumstances. The same was true of the upwardly mobile men, whose experience was no better than would be expected on the basis of their lifetime social circumstances (Hart et al, 1998).

A more sophisticated version of the social selection argument relates to intergenerational mobility, between the social location of the parental family and the social location of the individual, once they have left the parental home. Intergenerational selection could occur if childhood factors simultaneously influenced the achieved adulthood social position of people and their health in adulthood. Intergenerational selection can be divided into direct selection – which is said to occur if it is shown that health status in childhood determines both health status and socio-economic position in adulthood – and indirect selection – if common background factors such as childhood deprivation, height, education, etc determine both social mobility and later health (Davey Smith et al, 1994).

The evidence suggests that intergenerational selection does not contribute in a major way to socio-economic differentials in health among adults (Blane et al, 1993; Hart et al, 1998). Also, even if they were operating, these explanations should not necessarily be seen as 'health-related selection'. Such selection was initially formulated as a way in which social position and health become linked in the absence of a causal pathway from social environment to health. Many of the associations which could be interpreted as 'indirect selection' could equally be seen as reflecting the accumulation of social disadvantage. The 'background factors' postulated to be involved in such indirect selection are themselves the outcomes of social processes, so indirect selection is just one way in which disadvantage at one stage of life increases the probability of disadvantage at a later stage. If being ill in childhood makes people poor, you should ask why the poor were more likely to be ill when they were young.

Behavioural and cultural explanations

There is considerable interest in the possibility that health-related behaviours – particularly cigarette smoking, diet, lack of exercise and alcohol consumption – underlie inequalities in health. Several aspects of this approach must be considered, and we do this below. Firstly, does the social patterning of these behaviours match the social patterning of health and mortality? Secondly, how much do these behavioural differences account for the socio-economic differences in various health outcomes? Thirdly, should health-related behaviours simply be seen as a cause of health inequalities, or should they also be seen as an outcome of differences in the material circumstances between socio-economic groups?

Diet

We now consider the social patterning of diet and nutrient intake in some detail, as the impression that the diets of poor people (and those from the north) were a major cause of the poor health of these groups was propagated strongly (and insensitively) by some members of the last Conservative administration (Radical Statistics Health Group, 1987). Also we ask what the appropriate level for analysing and accounting for social class differences in diet should be. Should we think solely in terms of 'life-style choices' or should we consider the structural constraints on diet in different social groups? The results presented below are quite complex and we have tried to simplify them as much as possible, but this is the nature of work which considers proximal (generally biological) explanations for inequalities in health.

The 1986-87 dietary and nutritional survey of British adults (Gregory et al, 1990) provides some of the best data on socio-economic differentials in diet in Britain. In this study a representative sample of the adult population of England, Wales and Scotland, completed a seven-day weighed intake record. The results demonstrate a range of socio-economic differentials in dietary intake. Men in manual occupations reported higher intakes of dietary energy, presumably reflecting higher levels of physical activity. This finding has been seen elsewhere (Fehily et al, 1984). In contrast, women in non-manual occupations reported higher energy intakes than those in manual occupations. This may be an artefact of differential rates of dietary under-reporting according to social class (Pryer et al, 1995). Mean total and saturated fatty acid intakes, as a proportion of dietary energy, were not associated with social class in the British survey. These data are important as fat – in particular saturated fat – is considered to be the most important component of the diet that leads to coronary heart disease. The data suggest, therefore, that the amount of total and saturated dietary fat may not play a major role in the excess coronary risk among adults in less favourable social circumstances. This interpretation is supported by the findings (Braddon et al, 1988) of the National Survey of Health and Development (the 1946 birth cohort), from a seven-day diet diary completed in 1982, which show that saturated fatty acid intake did not vary by education level among men. Among women it was highest in those with university education (ie the reverse of what would be expected if saturated fat intake were the cause of high rates of disease in women with less education). Therefore, diet – in the main way it is currently believed to increase coronary heart disease risk – does not appear to contribute greatly to the direction or the trends in social class differentials in coronary heart disease. Evidence from other studies points to the same conclusion (Cade et al, 1998; Morgan et al, 1989).

Although fat intake appeared to be largely unassociated with social position among adults in the 1980s, the micronutrient density of the diet differed markedly by social class. Vitamins A, B and C, and iron, magnesium, potassium, calcium and phosphorus were all present at higher levels in the diets of those in higher social classes. Congruent findings have come from a study of nutrient intakes in lone-parent households (Dowler and Calvert, 1995). Intakes were compared for lone mothers in relation to whether they received Income Support or not. The average weekly income in households claiming Income Support was £87 in this study; for those not claiming Income Support it was £226 (Table 3.7). The large differentials in micronutrient density point to a social influence on food consumption patterns. In short, poor people are consuming less of the foodstuffs which are thought to be beneficial for health, but the differences presented in the table cannot plausibly account for the extent and range of socio-economic inequalities in health, although they may contribute to differences with respect to some health problems.

Table 3.7: Mean intakes of nutrients and intakes (% dietary reference values*) by Income Support (IS) receipt for UK female lone parents, London (1992-93) (n=126)

Nutrient	Mean IS (n=85)	SE	Mean No IS (n=41)	SE	Statistical significance of difference by ANOVA: P
Energy: Kcal	1,743	55	1,895	85	n/s
MJ	7.3	0.23	7.9	0.36	n/s
% EAR	8.4	2.8	88	3.6	n/s
Protein (% RNI)	144	4.8	154	7.4	n/s
Fat, total (g)	77	2.8	81	4.8	n/s
Iron (% RNI)	65	2.7	89	6.2	0.0001
Folate (% RNI)	90	4.3	107	7.4	0.032
Calcium (% RNI)	98	4.8	103	5.8	n/s
Zinc (% RNI)	107	4.4	118	6.8	n/s
Vitamin A (% RNI)	96	+	129	+	n/s
Vitamin C (% RNI)	94	+	155	+	0.005
Vitamin E (% safe intake)	162	+	206	+	0.018

Notes: Values are arithmetic mean of % dietary reference value, except for fat, with their standard errors. Geometric means are given for vitamins A, C and E. SE, standard error; RNI, reference nutrient intake; EAR, estimated average requirement. *DoH (1991). + No standard errors were presented; results were expressed as geometric means.

Source: Dowler and Calvert (1995)

Several studies demonstrate that those least able to purchase a healthy diet due to financial constraints are those most likely to be disadvantaged with regard to access to healthy micronutrient-dense food. Thus a shopping basket survey in Glasgow demonstrated that households in a less economically favoured area paid more for a healthy basket of food than households in a more favoured area, while there was no difference in the cost of an unhealthy basket of food. It was also noted that several items of the healthy food basket were simply not available in the less favoured area (Sooman et al, 1993). A similar survey was carried out in London in 1988 and repeated in 1995. At both times healthy food was more expensive in the deprived area, while unhealthy food was slightly cheaper in the deprived area (Lobstein, 1995). This study suggested that the situation for those living in the deprived area had become relatively worse between 1988 and 1995.

Poorer families have been disadvantaged by changes in food retailing. Between 1980 and 1992 the total number of food retail outlets in the country decreased by 35% (DoH, 1996). This reflects a decline in the number of small grocery retailers and specialist shops, including butchers and greengrocers, and an increase in large supermarkets. Such large retailers tend to be based outside of towns and customers require transport to reach them. The low rate of car ownership among poorer households makes it difficult for them to utilise these generally cheaper outlets. In essence the transfer of food retailing from smaller local retailers to large out-of-town superstores represents a transfer of costs from the food wholesaler – who is required to transport food to fewer outlets – to the customer, who must travel further to purchase food. This transfer represents a disproportionate burden to poorer households and contributes to widening inequalities in material circumstances. These trends have been widely documented (for example, see Wrigley, 1998).

Low-income households, residing in less affluent areas, are disadvantaged in other ways with respect to food, diet and nutrition. Such households may especially value the social resource represented by the personal nature of local shopping, given fewer alternative social opportunities. Shopping can become a demoralising experience for those whose choice is constrained by a lack of income (Dowler, 1996). The costs of cooking and of stocking essential items required for food preparation represent additional expenditure which may not be available in less well-off households. Dietary patterns cannot be thought of as simply reflecting 'life-style choices', with less healthy diets indicating less concern for health, ignorance or fecklessness. Instead, they are constrained by the social and economic circumstances in which people live.

Smoking

The current evidence on the distribution of health-related behaviours shows that these do match the distribution of health outcomes in some respects. Smoking by occupational social class has shown a strong gradient for some years and the relative differences between social classes has increased over this time. Figures 3.12 and 3.13 show data for men and women from 1974 to 1996. In the 1950s there were small (if any) socio-economic differences in smoking patterns, but these emerged in the 1960s, were marked by the 1970s, and became increasingly so over the 1980s and 1990s. It should be remembered that social class differences in all-cause mortality existed at a time when there was no gradient in smoking, or a reversed social class gradient – with higher smoking among the wealthier (Wald et al, 1988). Therefore, smoking patterns did not always mirror health differentials, and clearly could not explain such differentials during this earlier period. However, the increasing socio-economic gradient in smoking will certainly be a contributing factor to the increasing socio-economic differentials in mortality which have been seen over the past 40 years.

As with diet, we should consider smoking as an outcome of social processes, not simply as a reflection of individual choice, fecklessness or lack of knowledge regarding health consequences. For example, the work of Hilary Graham (Graham, 1995, 1996) demonstrates that smoking can be a rational choice for poor women whose lives are constrained by their lack of resources. When you have relatively little money, a packet of 10 cigarettes is a cheap pleasure in the short term and can easily be seen as a rational choice. In the long term, of course, cigarettes are very expensive in both financial and health terms, but the less money you have, the less sense it makes to consider the long term.

Exercise

The socio-economic distribution of exercise is complex. Manual occupational groups perform more exercise at work than do their non-manual peers, while leisure time exercise is more common among the more affluent social groups. This leads to an unclear picture with respect to total exercise performance. Table 3.8 shows the occupational social class differences in participation in sports, games and physical activities

Figure 3.12: **Percentage prevalence of cigarette smoking by occupational social class, men aged over 16, Britain (1974-96)**

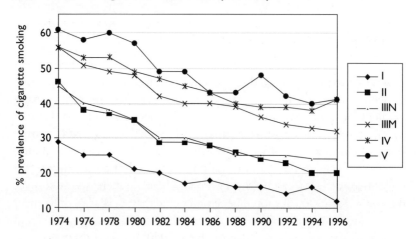

Source: Adapted from GHS (1996)

Figure 3.13: **Percentage prevalence of cigarette smoking by occupational social class, women aged over 16, Britain (1974-96)**

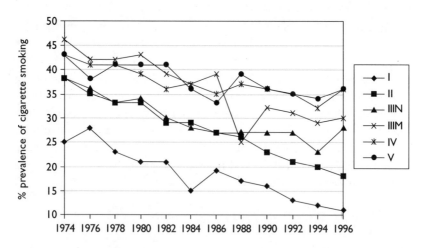

Source: Adapted from GHS (1996)

from the late 1980s to the late 1990s, showing very little change over this decade.

Table 3.8: **Trends in participation in sports, games and physical activities in the four weeks before interview by occupational social class, men and women (aged 16 and over, % participating), Britain (1987-96)**

Year	\multicolumn{7}{c}{Occupational social class}
	I	II	IIIN	IIIM	IV	V	Total
At least one activity (excluding walking)							
1987	65	52	45	48	34	26	45
1990	65	53	49	49	38	28	48
1993	64	53	49	46	36	31	47
1996	63	52	47	45	37	23	46
At least one activity							
1987	78	68	63	62	51	42	61
1990	79	71	67	66	55	46	65
1993	82	71	65	63	54	48	64
1996	80	69	66	63	55	45	64

Source: Adapted from GHS (1996)

Recent research on the health benefits of exercise have suggested that leisure time activity is protective against coronary heart disease and possibly some cancers, while occupational activity does not appear protective. This has been interpreted as reflecting the different nature of these two types of exercise, but it is equally likely that the different associations with health outcomes are generated by the fact that people who perform more exercise at work generally live in less favourable socio-economic environments and are at higher risk from unfavourable health outcomes because of this. Finally, participation in leisure time exercise is clearly influenced by the availability of good sports facilities (or pleasant residential areas for walking and jogging); both of these are more likely to be found in affluent than in deprived areas.

Health-related behaviours and socio-economic differentials in mortality

The contribution of health-related behaviours to socio-economic differences in mortality has been investigated in many studies. Well known among these is the Whitehall Study, discussed earlier. In this study smoking was more common among the lower grade civil servants.

However, large mortality differentials are seen for causes of death not considered to be smoking related (Figure 3.14). In subjects who never smoked, the mortality differentials were the same as in the whole cohort (Figure 3.15). While smoking is an important risk factor for death, it does not account for the socio-differentials in mortality in this study. Similar results have been found in various other cohort studies of this issue (eg Davey Smith et al, 1996a, 1996b, 1997).

The causes of the socio-economic gradient in coronary heart disease rates have been intensively investigated. Different smoking prevalences are considered particularly important in this regard (Baker et al, 1988). In an initial report from the British Regional Heart Study social class differences in smoking behaviour and blood pressure levels accounted for much of the socio-economic gradient (Pocock et al, 1987), although in a latter report this was no longer the case (Wannamethee and Shaper, 1997). The residual associations between social class and coronary heart disease incidence seen after adjustment for risk factors were suggested by Pocock and colleagues to be due to the inaccuracy inherent in using single measurements of risk factors as proxy measures of lifetime exposure and therefore to analyses not taking these risk factors fully into account. Imprecision in measurement of these factors renders the exploration of causes of differentials problematic (Davey Smith and Phillips, 1990). It is also the case that the use of social class alone leads to a marked underestimation of the strength of the relationship between socio-economic position and mortality, as the Longitudinal Study, among others, makes clear. In the Whitehall Study, the large differentials in cardiovascular (and all-cause) mortality by employment grade and car ownership could not be accounted for by differences in smoking, blood pressure, cholesterol, glucose intolerance, height or prevalent disease (Davey Smith et al, 1990a; Marmot et al, 1978). Similar results have been reported from other studies (Haan et al, 1987, 1989; Salonen, 1982; Holme et al, 1981; Buring et al, 1987; Hein et al, 1992; Davey Smith et al, 1996a, 1997; Davey Smith and Hart, 1998). The risk of mortality from many causes of death which have not been related to 'life-style' are also higher in less privileged groups (Najman and Congalton, 1979; Pearce et al, 1983; Marmot et al, 1984) which suggests that a wider range of explanatory factors should be explored.

Life circumstances: materialist explanations

The Black Report described as materialist those explanations emphasising hazards inherent in society. These are hazards to which some people have no choice but to be exposed given the present distribution of income and opportunity. In the light of the Black Report's stated preference for this type of explanation and the strong ecological correlations – presented in Chapter 2 – between material deprivation and both mortality and morbidity (see also Carstairs and Morris, 1989a, 1989b; Townsend et al, 1988) it is striking that it has been the subject of relatively little research during the past two decades. The health-damaging effects of physical exposures in certain occupations have long been recognised (Hunter, 1955) and recent research has demonstrated the additional importance of income (Wilkinson, 1989, 1990, 1992; Ecob and Davey Smith, 1999) and the possible role of psychosocial factors in this regard (Karasek et al, 1981; Alfredsson et al, 1985; Marmot and Theorell, 1989). Poor quality and/or damp housing have been shown to be associated with worse health and particularly with higher rates of respiratory disease in children (McCarthy et al, 1985; Martin et al, 1987; Platt et al, 1989; Lowry, 1989). There are thus many ways in which differences in life chances can be accounted for by differences in material well-being, but perhaps the best supported of these concern employment and income.

The men who were recorded as unemployed at the 1971 Census and also their wives were found to have a higher mortality rate than employed men and their wives (Moser et al, 1990). The relationship between income and health is well illustrated by an analysis of mortality risk among over 300,000 men in the 16 years following the screening for the Multiple Risk Factor Intervention Trial (Davey Smith et al, 1996a, 1996b). The age-adjusted relative rate of the poorest group of subjects was twice that of the richest group and the rate increased in a stepwise fashion between these extremes. The relative rates were further adjusted for differences between income groups in cigarette smoking, blood pressure, serum cholesterol, prevalent heart disease and diabetes. In consequence, the relative rate of the poorest group compared to the richest fell slightly but the stepwise progression between the extremes remained. When cardiovascular disease mortality, cancer mortality and death from the group of all other causes were analysed separately, differentials of similar magnitude, together with the same stepwise progression between the extremes, remained.

We discussed earlier the interest in the possible consequences of deprivation in early life for health in adulthood. Studies have suggested that cardiovascular and respiratory disease may have their origins in adverse conditions during development (Forsdahl, 1977, 1978; Barker and Osmond, 1986; Kaplan and Salonen, 1990; Davey Smith et al, 1998c).

Differential degrees of deprivation in childhood will therefore contribute to inequalities in health in later life.

Figure 3.14: **Mortality from causes of death unrelated to smoking, by employment grade and car ownership in the Whitehall Study of London civil servants (1967-80)**

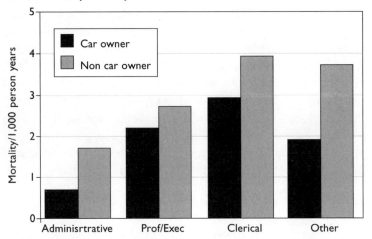

Source: Davey Smith et al (1994)

Figure 3.15: **All-cause mortality by employment grade and car ownership among participants who had never smoked in the Whitehall Study of London civil servants (1967-80)**

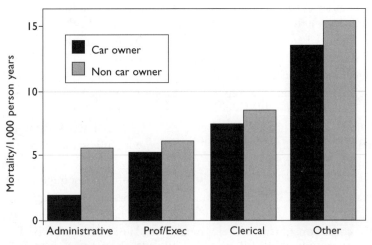

Source: Davey Smith et al (1994)

Each directly material factor (eg occupational hazards, poor housing, unemployment, childhood deprivation and so forth) may on its own make a modest contribution to the total socio-economic gradient in health. The modest size of these individual contributions can appear inconsistent with the powerful effect of the influence of such factors, as indicated by area deprivation correlations and the stepwise relationship between income and mortality. However, as we have discussed earlier, the form of social organisation we live under leads to the clustering of advantage or disadvantage over time and place. A woman in a low-income household is more likely to have been poorly nourished during her childhood, to herself be poorly nourished during pregnancy and therefore to produce a low birth weight or premature baby. This child, growing up in a low-income household, is in turn more likely to be disadvantaged in terms of diet, overcrowding, safe areas in which to play and opportunities for educational achievement. In such circumstances, growth and the development of health potential during childhood may be constrained. An adolescent from a low-income household is more likely to leave education at the minimum school-leaving age, with few qualifications and to experience unemployment before entering a low-paid, insecure and hazardous occupation with, for instance, no sick pay, poor holiday entitlements and no occupational pension scheme. An adult working in this sector of the labour market is more likely to experience periods of unemployment, to raise a family in financially difficult circumstances and to become permanently sick or retire early because their prematurely expended health can no longer cope with the physical demands of their work. A retired person who does not have an occupational pension is more likely to experience financial deprivation in the years leading up to their death. Throughout their lives people with these disadvantages are also likely to live in areas with characteristics which have an unfavourable effect on health.

By such mechanisms advantage and disadvantage cluster across the life-course. Although epidemiological evidence suggests that each of these factors individually could make only a modest contribution to total mortality, overall social class gradients in health can be explained in materialist terms by the accumulation of multiple factors over the course of life. Furthermore, the coexistence of a series of exposures within one person's life may generate greater health problems than would be anticipated from the known effect of single exposures. For example, the combination of an occupational exposure (arsenic or asbestos) and smoking generates a greater risk of lung cancer than would be expected from the simple addition of the known effects of the exposures experienced on their own (Hertz-Picciotto et al, 1992; Erren et al, 1999). This synergistic effect of combined exposures would contribute to the poor health outcomes of people who experience disadvantage in several components of their lives.

Our discussion of the process might suggest an all or nothing phenomenon in which individuals are either advantaged or disadvantaged. More accurately, the social structure is characterised by finely graded scale of advantage and disadvantage, with individuals differing in terms of the length and level of their exposure to a particular factor and in terms of the number of factors to which they are exposed. The 'fine grain' of socio-economic differentials in health parallels the fine grading of the social structure and of people's cumulative experience across their lives.

Research in this area has not advanced greatly since the appearance of the Black Report (DHSS, 1980; Townsend and Davidson, 1988; Davey Smith et al, 1990b; Blane et al, 1997). In that Report there is a sense of acceptance of a materialist explanation by a process of elimination: since the other explanations do not appear adequate, the remaining alternative is accepted. What is required is further research which determines the precise routes through which material disadvantage causes poor health. At the same time it should be recognised that a major reason for the relative paucity of evidence concerning the link between material conditions and health is the lack of enthusiasm for investigating this area among much of the research establishment (Blane, 1985; Blane et al, 1997).

Inequalities in health: one or many causes?

Much of the literature on health inequalities has dealt with all-cause mortality or general health measures, such as reports of long-standing illness or self-rated health. Even studies which have moved from such overall measures to more specific ones have tended to use a few broad categories of causes of death or forms of ill-health (Wannamethee and Shaper, 1997). Some investigators have hypothesised that there is a heightened general susceptibility to disease among groups in adverse socio-economic circumstances (Najman and Congalton, 1979; Marmot et al, 1984; Syme and Berkman, 1976; Susser et al, 1985). A wide variety of factors – psychosocial stress, poor diet, inadequate coping resources, genetic differences – have been advanced as the phenomenon underlying this heightened susceptibility (Valkonen, 1987; Thurlow, 1967; Najman,

1980) and putative physiological mechanisms, such as suppression of the immune system, have been discussed (Sterling and Eyer, 1981; Totman, 1987).

Examination of the socio-economic distribution of particular cancers, however, reveals wide heterogeneity in the strength and direction of associations (Davey Smith et al, 1991), which gives little support for theories of general susceptibility. A similar conclusion comes from the examination of the distribution of other causes of death (Davey Smith et al, 1996a, 1996b). It would appear that the theory of general susceptibility needs to be modified to integrate processes of specific aetiology (causes). Attempts to account for social class differences in health might be usefully conceptualised in terms of the balance between general susceptibility and specific aetiology, with consideration being given to which aspect of the relationship is being influenced by any one explanatory variable. Inequalities in overall health status result from the fact that it tends to be the important causes of ill-health, for example, coronary heart disease, stroke, lung cancer and respiratory disease, which show the largest socio-economic differentials. The social processes which concentrate the exposures, which increase the risk of these diseases on particular disadvantaged groups, therefore underlie health inequalities. Thus while 'general susceptibility' may not exist as a biological phenomenon there is certainly a social mechanism which damages the overall health status of those in the least favouable socio-economic situations.

Another useful way to think about inequalities in health is to consider them against the background of broad secular changes and international differences in health status and mortality risk. Over the 20th century, there have been very sizeable declines in mortality in most industrialised countries with, for example, infant mortality rates in the 1990s being only 5% of those at the turn of the century in England and Wales. For one to four-year-olds, the situation is even more dramatic – mortality rates for the 1990s are 2% of those at the turn of the century. Even among the middle-aged there have been substantial reductions, with end of the 20th century mortality rates being around one fifth to one third the rates seen at the beginning of the century (Charlton and Murphy, 1997). It is likely that the factors which have contributed to the sizeable reductions in mortality are also those which contribute to the current differentials in mortality between socio-economic groups.

If our understanding of the factors generating socio-economic differentials in health is to be advanced we need to consider the particular factors which contribute to international differences, secular trends and socio-economic differentials, in particular causes of ill-health. Some illustrative cases are given here. Internationally, stomach cancer is a major cause of mortality, being one of the most common cancers seen in developing countries and in earlier times in developed countries. Stroke mortality shows a similar geographical and temporal distribution to stomach cancer mortality and also has declined dramatically over this century. Among middle-aged men and women in England and Wales, stroke mortality at the beginning of the 20th century was seven times higher than at the end of the century (Charlton and Murphy, 1997). The declines in stroke and stomach cancer in England and Wales contributed to the declines in overall mortality among post-childhood age groups. The risk of these diseases seems to be established to a sizeable extent in childhood. People migrating from high to low stomach cancer areas after childhood take with them the risk of stomach cancer of the place they have migrated from (Coggon et al, 1990). The existence of cohort effects – such that people born in each successive period have lower mortality than those from a previous period – support this conclusion (Hansson et al, 1991).

Data from the West of Scotland Collaborative Study (Davey Smith et al, 1998d) demonstrate that stomach cancer and stroke risk is associated with parental socio-economic position – and hence a person's circumstances in childhood – more strongly than to their social position in adult life. It is suggested that the material conditions of existence at the time people who are currently dying of stomach cancer and stroke were born are important factors underlying current risk for these conditions. Adverse socio-economic circumstances in childhood favour the acquisition of infection with the bacteria *Helicobacter pylori* (Mendall et al, 1992) and infection appears to be an important cause of stomach cancer. Declining rates of *Helicobacter pylori* infection have accompanied improving social conditions over the century and thus may underlie the falling rates of stomach cancer mortality. Infections acquired in childhood may also be important factors in the production of risk of stroke in adult life. Thus, current morbidity and mortality patterns for these conditions could be related directly to poverty-associated factors such as overcrowding and hygiene practices – that influence acquisition of infections – acting in early life.

For other important causes of morbidity and mortality in adulthood, socially-patterned exposures acting in early life appear to interact with or accumulate with later life exposures. Thus, morbidity and mortality from respiratory disease in adulthood are related to housing conditions and infections acquired in childhood. Smoking and occupational exposures in later life then influence disease risk, in association with these earlier life factors (Mann et al, 1992). In the case of diabetes, hypertension and coronary heart disease, low birth weight – which is strongly socially-patterned and related to intergenerational experiences as well as maternal nutrition – interacts with obesity in later life (increasingly prevalent among people in unfavourable social circumstances) to produce elevated disease risk (Phillips et al, 1994; Leon et al, 1996; Frankel et al, 1996; Lithell et al, 1996). Large differences in relative and absolute risk for various forms of morbidity can be demonstrated when groups are defined by clusters of socially-patterned adverse exposures acting throughout life. These exposures include health-related behaviours and the effects of psychosocial exposures such as job insecurity, as well as the direct influences of material circumstances.

Conclusion

The evidence on the causes of health inequalities demonstrate that they are not due to any simple or singular explanation – less favourable profiles of health-related behaviours among the deprived; or the fact that the sick are more likely to become poor, for example. We also see that some of the factors which contribute to health inequalities – such as smoking and inadequate diet – are themselves strongly influenced by the unequal distribution of income, wealth and life chances in general. These factors do not simply reflect the lack of knowledge or fecklessness of the poorer members of society. If we are to tackle inequalities in health we need an approach which deals with the fundamental causes of such inequalities, not one which focuses mainly on those processes which mediate between social disadvantage and poor health.

An approach aimed at the underlying causes of health inequalities has greater potential for producing meaningful changes in health and such an approach will not simply substitute one set of poor health outcomes for another. In this regard it is important to remember that health inequalities have persisted over a period when the major causes of ill-health and death have changed dramatically. Since different exposures are responsible for these different causes of death it is clear that with the continued existence of poverty and inequality, those living in less advantaged social circumstances receive the worst end of the deal whatever the actual diseases and the set of exposures which mediate between social disadvantage and disease are. Over the years those who are now elderly and who have been living in the poorest households will have been more exposed to impure water, inadequate sewerage, overcrowding, damp housing, inadequate diet, job insecurity, smoking and lack of exercise. Thus the inequalities in health have persisted over a time when infectious diseases have ceased to be the major cause of death, because inequalities in infectious diseases have been superseded by inequalities in chronic diseases.

Given our understanding of the manner by which social disadvantage translates into poor health we can identify those periods of the life-course when people are particularly vulnerable to the effects of adverse social circumstances. In Box 3.1 we list these 'critical periods' (adapted from Bartley et al, 1997) when the absence of resources can lead to unfavourable effects which damage health or reduce quality of life. At some stages the lack of such resources can lead to life trajectories which increase the likelihood of encountering more disadvantage. There are, therefore, 'multiplier effects' – such that even relatively small differences in social circumstances are magnified by later events (which are in part set in train by these earlier experiences). Policies aimed at reducing inequalities in health need to pay particular attention to these 'critical periods' (see Box 3.1), as well as overall inequality, and need to be designed to avoid social disadvantage being entrained by such a 'multiplier effect'. Most importantly, to be successful, such policies must be aimed at the fundamental causes of inequality, rather than solely at some of the intermediary processes in this chain.

Box 3.1: 'Critical periods' of the life-course

- Fetal development
- Birth
- Nutrition, growth and health in childhood
- Educational career
- Leaving parental home
- Entering labour market
- Establishing social and sexual relationships
- Job loss or insecurity
- Parenthood
- Episodes of illness
- Labour market exit
- Chronic sickness
- Loss of full independence

Source: Adapted from Bartley et al (1997)

FOUR

The widening gap

Summary

There is evidence that the health gap is widening and that this widening has followed socio-economic polarisation in Britain. As the poor have become relatively poorer and have become concentrated into particular areas of the country, poor health has similarly become more concentrated both by social group and by area over the last 20 years.

- Although infant mortality is falling overall, social class differences in infant mortality are clear and are widening. Babies born into poor families are increasingly disadvantaged.

- The life expectancy gap between social classes is widening and this is not due to changes in social class sizes.

- Geographical differences in mortality are widening and in relative terms are now larger than ever measured before. The recent growth in area inequalities began around 1980.

- These widening gaps are real and cannot be attributed to measurement issues or statistical biases. They have real, lethal, meaning for large groups of people living in Britain today.

Over the past two decades, the widening gap in health has been anticipated by a widening gap in terms of a number of other socio-economic measures of well-being:

- *Income:* the poorest 10% of single adult households were, on average, £208 per year worse off in 1995/96 than in 1979; the richest 10% became £6,968 per year richer in real terms.

- *Poverty:* the proportion of households living at below half average income increased from less than 8% in 1977/78 to 24% in 1995/96.

- *Wealth:* the distribution of wealth in the UK hardly changed between 1983 and 1994. The most wealthy 1% have consistently owned around 20% of the total marketable wealth.

- *Unemployment:* between 1981 and 1991 unemployment and underemployment grew fastest in the areas of Britain which now have the worst and worsening health.

Introduction

Chapter 2 has established that there is a very wide health gap in Britain, and Chapter 3 has demonstrated that this gap can *primarily* be explained by social and economic disadvantage, especially poverty, and that the effects of such disadvantage accumulate through the life-course. This chapter presents evidence of a *widening gap* in Britain, in terms of health, but also in terms of social and economic indicators. The most important factor is an increased proportion of the population living in relative poverty and there being greater income inequality overall. It is surely no coincidence that these processes have occurred concurrently over the past two decades.

In order to consider changes over time, comparative measures are needed – geographical boundaries need to be frozen, definitions of measures, such as unemployment, need to be consistent, and so on. This limits the amount of data that are available (see Dorling, 1995 for more details). However, the most robust evidence available is presented here to show both that the health gap is widening and that this widening is a result of widening inequalities in other aspects of life in Britain over time.

The widening gap between communities

Mortality rates have polarised between communities since the early 1980s. We can see this most clearly when we compare communities over time according to their average level of income. Figure 4.1 illustrates the long history of studies such as this – showing how in the 1930s in Stockton-on-Tees income differences produced large differences in death rates. Such studies can now be brought up to date, and conducted nationally. With estimates of the 1991 individual households' income calculated for Chapter 2 we have divided the 641 parliamentary constituencies of Britain into 10 equal-sized population groups so that here we can compare the same set of constituencies at each point in time. These are decile groups of the population according to the average incomes of people living in their constituencies (see Table 2.12 and the accompanying text for further explanations). In the poorest 10% of constituencies, average incomes of people in the workforce were £9,785 per year in 1991 and £3,700 higher in the richest 10% of constituencies. Although this difference may look small it has a very significant effect on the lives of the people living in these areas. When the average income in large communities is less than £200 per week (as it is in the poorest areas), a few extra pounds a week would make a great deal of difference to people's everyday lives. The lack of this money leads to the loss of many opportunities. This effect can be seen directly – from an inability to buy the goods and services that most people would consider to be necessities (such as being able to heat your home) as well as indirectly (such as through limiting aspirations) – resulting in thousands of premature deaths per year in these areas.

Figure 4.1: Relation between incomes and death rates, Stockton-on-Tees (1930s)

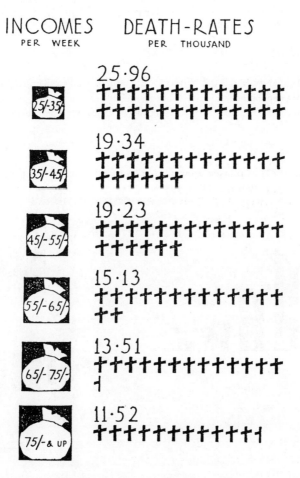

Note: Incomes are shillings per week (1930s prices)
Source: M'Gonigle and Kirby (1936)

Table 4.1: SMRs for deaths under 65 by constituencies grouped by income in 1991, Britain (1981-95)

Decile area	Average income 1991	SMRs of population aged under 65			
		1981-85	1986-90	1991-95	Change*
1	£9,785	127	131	134	+8
2	£10,508	118	119	120	+2
3	£10,904	110	110	108	-2
4	£11,200	103	104	101	-2
5	£11,446	101	100	100	-1
6	£11,728	99	99	97	-2
7	£12,039	94	93	90	-4
8	£12,330	89	87	84	-4
9	£12,744	87	86	83	-4
10	£13,485	84	81	80	-4

Note: England and Wales SMR = 100 at each time period to maintain consistency with official and published series. *Change is absolute percentage point change between 1981-85 and 1991-95, due to rounding decile 1 change is +8 percentage points not +7.
Source: Analysis by authors

Figure 4.2: SMRs of people aged under 65 by constituencies grouped by income in 1991, Britain (1981-95)

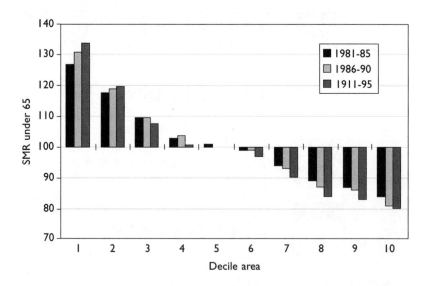

Note: England and Wales SMR = 100 at each time period.
Source: Analysis by authors

Table 4.1 and Figure 4.2 show that, in the early 1980s, the mortality rate in the 10% of constituencies with the lowest incomes was 27% above the average for Britain, but was 34% above the average just 10 years later and so the health gap has grown. In the poorest income areas of Britain people aged under 65 are a third more likely to die each year than is the population as a whole. Ten years ago, the equivalent figure was just over a quarter more likely. In the richest areas, only 80 people die for every 100 nationally, 4% fewer than 10 years ago. The geographical gap is wider for men than for women. The gap has been getting rapidly wider for men. The gap is growing for women as well, but not as quickly, as can be seen from Table 4.2 and Figure 4.3. It is important to point out that here we are always comparing the same places, defined according to average incomes in 1991.

Table 4.2: **SMRs by constituencies grouped by income in 1991, for men and for women, Britain (1981-95)**

	SMR under 65: Men				SMR under 65: Women			
Decile area	1981-85	1986-90	1991-95	Change	1981-85	1986-90	1991-95	Change
1	128	133	137	9	125	129	130	5
2	118	120	121	3	118	118	119	1
3	110	110	108	-2	110	108	108	-2
4	104	103	101	-3	103	104	102	-1
5	101	100	99	-2	100	100	101	1
6	99	99	97	-2	99	99	98	-1
7	94	93	90	-3	94	93	90	-4
8	88	87	83	-5	90	88	87	-3
9	86	85	82	-4	88	87	86	-2
10	83	80	79	-3	86	83	81	-5

Note: Deciles are arranged in increasing order of average incomes.
Source: Analysis by authors, see Table 4.1

Figure 4.3: Change in SMRs by constituencies grouped by income in 1991, for men and for women, Britain (1981-95)

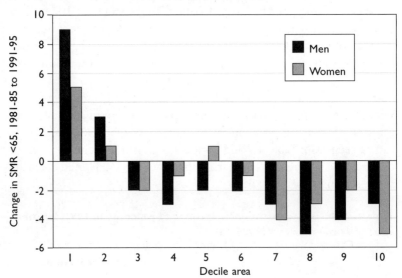

Source: Table 4.2

The historical gap between communities

Is this widening gap part of a long-term trend of increasing health inequality? It could be argued that, as mortality rates fall in general, we should expect the gap to grow as it is usually the rich who benefit first from any improvement in living standards. To test this hypothesis, we need to consider a longer period of time than the 1980s and 1990s and see how the most recent trends in inequality compare to trends in a longer historical series.

Before 1981 (at least in England and Wales) mortality statistics were only available in printed form and these were only published for particular areas used by the Registrar General in the government's Decennial Supplement on mortality. Different areas were used in Scotland. There were 292 of these areas in Britain and they consisted largely of London boroughs, metropolitan boroughs, the urban districts of counties, the rural remainders of counties, Scottish Burghs, Islands and Scottish Counties. The boundaries of these areas were all defined prior to the 1974 reorganisation of local government. Over such a long period of time no independent measure of socio-economic position, such as average incomes, is available and so instead a comparison has to be made between the worst off (in terms of health) at one time period with the worst off (in terms of health) now.

In Table 4.3, contemporary mortality ratios have been calculated using the individual postcoded mortality records. This process is described further in the Joseph Rowntree Foundation report *Death in Britain* (Dorling, 1997). Those statistics are reproduced here with added data for the most recent years available: 1993-95. They are shown graphically in Figure 4.4 which illustrates how inequalities have widened over time.

The figures in Table 4.3 differ from those in Tables 4.1 and 4.2 for two reasons. Firstly, although the areas still contain tenths of the population, they are groupings of different types of areas as described above (old county boroughs rather than modern constituencies). Secondly, the areas are sorted by mortality ratios rather than income so the gap shown is wider, but the historical comparability is still valid. The table shows that, in general, inequalities in mortality have increased over time, but that this has not always been the case. Most importantly, inequalities in mortality decreased between 1963 and 1969. Since then, they have increased, but only rapidly since 1981. We do not have the data needed to know exactly whether this increase began in, say 1977, 1979 or 1981. Regardless of when the process began, inequalities in mortality now stand at the highest levels ever recorded. People living in the worst mortality decile (of historically comparable areas) between 1993 and 1995 were 47% more likely to die in any year before the age of 65 as compared to the national average.

Table 4.3: **Age-sex SMR for deaths under 65 in Britain by deciles of population (grouped by old county borough and ordered by SMR), Britain (1950-95)**

Decile	1950-53	1959-63	1969-73	1981-85	1986-89	1990-92	1993-95
1	131.0	135.5	131.2	135.0	139.2	142.3	147.4
2	118.1	123.0	115.6	118.6	120.9	121.4	120.9
3	112.1	116.5	112.0	114.2	113.9	111.3	112.7
4	107.0	110.7	108.1	109.8	106.9	104.9	106.7
5	102.5	104.5	103.0	102.1	102.2	99.0	98.5
6	98.6	97.4	96.9	95.7	95.6	93.5	94.6
7	93.1	90.9	91.8	91.6	91.9	90.9	91.7
8	88.7	87.6	88.9	89.3	89.1	86.5	86.6
9	85.7	83.1	87.0	84.3	83.0	80.4	80.2
10	81.8	77.1	83.0	79.2	78.1	76.2	74.5
Ratio 10:1	1.60	1.75	1.58	1.70	1.78	1.87	1.98

Source: Analysis by authors; see Dorling (1997) for more details

Figure 4.4: **Age-sex SMR for deaths under 65 in Britain by deciles of population (grouped by old county borough and ordered by SMR), Britain (1950-95)**

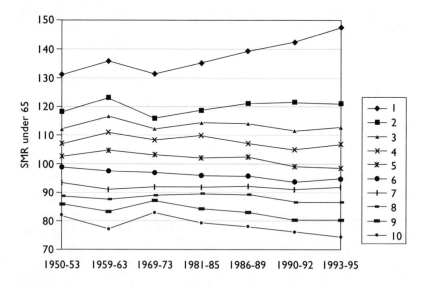

Source: Table 4.3

The last row of Table 4.3 ('ratio 10:1') shows that inequalities in mortality between areas rose in the 1950s then fell during the 1960s and stayed low in the 1970s. Before the early 1980s, the highest ratio recorded was around the 1961 Census – towards the end of 13 years of Conservative rule. The ratio of inequality fell most rapidly during the 1964-70 Wilson administration and did not rise back to its 1961 levels under the Heath or Callaghan administrations. It was only under the leadership of Mrs Thatcher that the ratio managed to rise to over 1.8, to end up, under John Major, at almost 2.0. Why was the political trend apparently reflected? Why do inequalities in mortality tend to rise when the Conservative Party has been in power? Table 4.4 gives some clues as it shows these ratios of health inequality compared to the proportion of the population living below half average incomes at these times. Although, given the discussion in Chapter 3, we would expect there to be time lags between income and health inequality (for instance, see the last time period in Figure 4.5 where income inequality was stable but mortality inequalities continued to increase). However, for younger age groups and for more direct causes of death (such as suicides rates related to unemployment levels) time lags can be very short. It is also important to realise that even persistent stable social inequalities may lead to rising inequalities in health as their influence accumulates over time.

Figure 4.5: Inequality ratios of SMRs for deaths under 65 in Britain and % of households below half average income (HBAI) (1950-95)

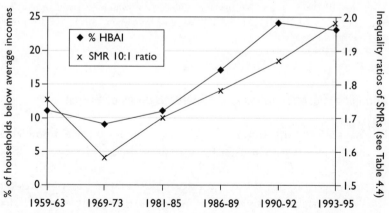

Note: No HBAI figures are available for 1950-53; the minimum estimate has been taken for each period; SMR data are only available for certain years before 1981 from the Decennial Reviews.

Source: DSS (1998a)

Table 4.4 and Figure 4.5 show that inequalities in mortality were lowest in Britain when inequalities in income were lowest – between 1969 and 1973 – following the Labour governments of 1964-70. Inequalities in income reached their minimum in 1977 but no comparable data on mortality in 1977 by area are available. This is partly because the new Conservative government of 1979 introduced severe cuts to the (then) Office of Population Censuses and Surveys and partly because of the reorganisation of local government districts in 1974 breaking the historical series of mortality data by area. Whether the trend changed in 1977, 1979 or 1981, what matters is the change after 1981. It was only in the 1980s that both inequalities in health and inequalities in income rose dramatically, rose together and rose to unprecedented levels. Both levels of inequality had fallen together before (between 1963 and 1969, see Figure 4.5). Reductions in health inequalities are thus achievable even in a short space of time, but they have only occurred when there has also been a reduction in income inequalities.

Table 4.4: Inequality ratios of SMRs for deaths under 65 in Britain and % of households below half average income (HBAI) (1950-95)

Decile	1950-53	1959-63	1969-73	1981-85	1986-89	1990-92	1993-95
Ratio 10:1	1.60	1.75	1.58	1.70	1.78	1.87	1.98
HBAI (%)	-	11	9	11	17	24	23

Note: No HBAI figures are available for 1950-53; the minimum estimate has been taken for each period; SMR data are only available for certain years before 1981 from the Decennial Reviews.
Source: DSS (1998a) and Table 4.3

Changing mortality ratios in the extreme areas of Britain

In Chapter 2 the situation in the 28 constituencies at the extreme ends of the health inequalities scale was described. How were these constituencies affected by the dramatic rise in income and social inequality during the 1980s and early 1990s? Table 4.5 compares the 1991-95 mortality ratios in these areas with the equivalent ratios for 1981-85.

Mortality ratios rose from 155 to 178 in the 'worst health' areas; at the same time they fell from 76 to 68 in the 'best health' areas. The ratio of inequality between these two extreme parts of Britain rose from 2.1 to 2.6 over 10 years. A rise in inequality is not surprising as these areas were chosen for study because they had the most extreme ratios in the latter period, but the extent of the rise is striking. Tables 4.3 and 4.4 showing income inequality and trends over time from 1950-95 confirm that this rise is unlikely to be an artefact of the specific selection of these areas. Rather, these areas are indicative of what happened across Britain during the 1980s, although we are showing some of the most extreme changes by concentrating on the extreme areas.

Table 4.5 shows that mortality has become more concentrated spatially, as is highlighted by considering deciles of the population. In terms of health the table looks at the current 'best health' and 'worst health' million adults aged under 65. The table shows that the SMRs for the 'worst health' million, which were twice as high a decade ago compared to those for the 'best health' million, are now 2.6 times as high. The first row of the table shows that the SMRs (which were 79 points higher in the 1980s) rose to be 110 points higher in the 1990s when the two sets of areas are contrasted. The SMR for all of Britain has fallen from 102 to 100 (using England and Wales as 100) as rates in Scotland as a whole have fallen and are now in line with England and Wales. The increase in SMRs for the 'worst health' million is almost three times greater than the decrease for the 'best health' million. The table also shows that almost all constituencies in the 'worst health' areas have lost population aged under 65 – mainly due to out-migration (totalling 56,000 people in 10 years) whereas the 'best health' areas have gained 82,000. For those who did not leave these areas, had the mortality gap not widened, then 11% of people who died between 1991 and 1995 in the 'worst health' areas would not have died. For all of Britain, 7% of all deaths in this age group would not have occurred if *just* the improvements in mortality rates enjoyed by the 'best health' million been enjoyed by all. Had the low levels of mortality that the 'best health' million experience been enjoyed by all, then very many more would not have died (see Chapter 2). The situation is getting worse. In absolute terms the extent of this worsening can be seen in the additional unnecessary premature deaths of the thousands of people who have died young in Britain between 1991 and 1995.

Table 4.5: Constituencies where people are most at risk of premature death in Britain 1991-95 – SMR change since 1981-85

		SMR<65				
Rank	**Name**	**SMR 1981-85**	**SMR 1991-95**	**SMR change**	**Pop<65 change**	**Avoidable change %**
'Worst health' less 'best health' areas		**+79**	**+110**	**+31**	**-138,248**	**+11**
1	Glasgow Shettleston	184	234	50	-1,719	12
2	Glasgow Springburn	177	217	39	-9,481	11
3	Glasgow Maryhill	163	196	33	-1,139	12
4	Glasgow Pollok	155	187	31	-10,022	12
5	Glasgow Anniesland	150	181	32	-9,325	13
6	Glasgow Baillieston	152	180	29	-11,728	12
7	Manchester Central	166	173	7	-1,931	6
8	Glasgow Govan	146	172	26	330	12
9	Liverpool Riverside	155	172	16	-7,638	9
10	Manchester Blackley	147	169	22	-501	11
11	Greenock and Inverclyde	148	164	17	-6,485	10
12	Salford	154	163	9	-6,819	8
13	Tyne Bridge	148	158	10	-3,395	8
14	Glasgow Kelvin	156	158	2	3,200	6
15	Southwark North and Bermondsey	123	156	33	10,783	18
'Worst health' million		*155*	*178*	*23*	*-55,869*	*11*
Rank	**Name**					
1	Wokingham	71	65	-6	17,926	
2	Woodspring	73	65	-8	4,490	
3	Romsey	76	65	-11	5,343	
4	Sheffield Hallam	78	66	-12	3,183	
5	South Cambridgeshire	70	66	-3	6,961	
6	Chesham and Amersham	71	67	-3	-868	
7	South Norfolk	77	69	-8	6,708	
8	West Chelmsford	78	69	-9	5,473	
9	South Suffolk	85	69	-16	3,882	
10	Witney	73	69	-3	9,024	
11	Esher and Walton	74	69	-4	4,649	
12	Northavon	76	70	-6	7,327	
13	Buckingham	86	71	-15	8,281	
'Best health' million		*76*	*68*	*-8*	*82,379*	
Britain		**102***	**100**	**-2**	**1,713,830**	**7**

Notes: Avoidable deaths are those deaths which would not have occurred had the mortality rate of the 'best health' million been experienced by everybody living in Britain during each time period. The population of each constituency is estimated for 1993 from the Estimating with Confidence Project ward statistics updated by the 1996 ONS age/sex mid-year estimates of population for local authority districts. The 1983 population estimates are from this and the 1981 Census of population. The mortality numbers are assigned to constituencies through the postcodes of the deceased (see Dorling, 1997). *The SMR for Britain in 1981-85 is 102 because throughout this book SMRs are calculated with the rate set to 100 for England and Wales. During 1991 to 1995 overall mortality rates in Scotland fell to the British average.

Source: Analysis by authors

Figure 4.6: **Change in premature death ratios in the extreme areas of Britain, 1981-85 to 1991-95**

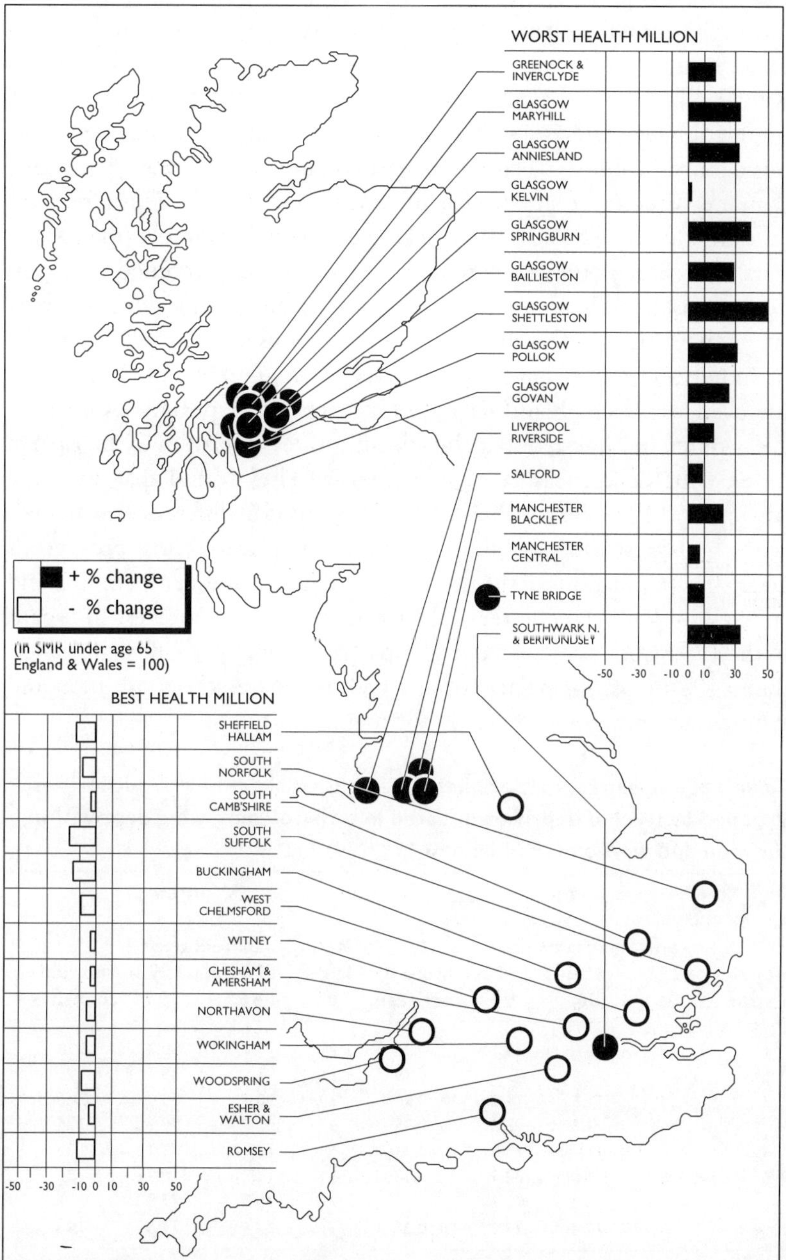

Source: Table 4.5

Figure 4.6 maps these changes in SMRs in the 'best' and 'worst' health areas we have been following through this book. The map illustrates that there is a great deal of local variability in the changes in mortality ratios, although they have all risen in the 'worst health' areas and have all fallen in the 'best health' areas. The smallest rise occurred in Glasgow Kelvin, which, as mentioned several times in Chapter 2, is an area whose population characteristics are changing rapidly (this was indicated by its population profile). Measures of change are almost always less stable than measures of the situation at any one period of time. This is because random fluctuations can effect change statistics far more than static statistics. This is the main reason why we have combined the areas being considered here – so that the statistics which we present are robust when they concern the changing fates of groups of one million people.

Other researchers have also reported a geographical polarisation in life chances. Raleigh and Kiri (1997) report life expectancies for men and women in English district health authorities in relation to the Jarman index which is a measure of deprivation. They found that, over the time period 1984-86 to 1992-94, the geographical differences widened, with the largest gains in life expectancy being in the most prosperous areas. The populations of the most deprived health authorities in England (inner London, Manchester and Liverpool) had the shortest life spans in the 1980s and experienced negligible improvements in life expectancy. Table 4.6 shows this polarisation, which is apparent for both men and women, but much more clearly for men.

Table 4.6: Life expectancy at birth for English district health authorities grouped by level of deprivation, listed in order of increasing deprivation, for men and women (1984-86 and 1992-94)

| Level of deprivation | Men Life | | | | Women Life | | | |
	Rank 1984-86	expectancy 1984-86	1992-94	% annual increase	Rank 1984-86	expectancy 1984-86	1992-94	% annual increase
1	1	73.0	75.2	0.38	2	78.4	80.2	0.28
2	2	72.9	75.0	0.35	1	78.5	80.1	0.25
3	3	72.6	74.8	0.36	3	78.4	80.0	0.25
4	4	71.6	73.7	0.35	4	77.6	79.1	0.24
5	5	71.1	73.0	0.34	6	77.1	78.7	0.25
6	6	71.0	72.9	0.32	5	77.3	78.9	0.26
7	7	70.2	71.2	0.18	7	76.8	77.8	0.17
England		**72.1**	**74.1**	**0.35**		**77.9**	**79.5**	**0.25**

Note: Rank 7 is the highest level of deprivation
Source: Adapted from Raleigh and Kiri (1997)

Geographical polarisation by age groups

The uneven distribution of improvements in life expectancy can also be seen when specific age groups are considered. Although smaller numbers of deaths are being looked at, the statistics are nonetheless both robust and meaningful for the million people aggregated into the 'worst' and 'best' health constituencies. For Britain as a whole, mortality rates have decreased for all the age groups shown in Table 4.7. For the 'worst health' million, however, they have actually *increased* in real terms (by 7%) for young adults aged 15-44. The slight improvement seen for infants, children and older age groups are all much less than the improvements experienced by the 'best health' million people in these same age groups. The improvements in mortality rates for infants in the 'best health' areas are twice as large as for infants in the 'worst health' areas. For children aged one to four, the 'best health' areas have seen improvements 10 times as great as in the 'worst health' areas. The health gap is growing for all age groups and for young adults this translates into more premature deaths in absolute terms in the 'worst health' areas of Britain.

Figure 4.7 maps the absolute polarisation in life chances seen for adults aged 15-44 in the extreme areas of Britain. In all the 'best health' areas mortality rates fell for this age group over the 10 years 1981-85 to 1991-95. Many of these falls were very large. In contrast, mortality rates rose in *absolute* terms in 10 of the 15 'worst health' areas of the country for young adults. The largest increase was a 44% rise in Southwark North and Bermondsey. These are all increases in mortality from an already very high level. It is also still important to remember that change statistics are more variable than the rates calculated at any particular time, but the overall increase of 7% is a true indicator of how young adults' life chances have deteriorated absolutely over the 1980s and early 1990s in the 'worst health' areas of Britain.

The widening health gap by cause of death – coronary heart disease

Table 4.8 below uses the same population deciles as those in Table 4.3 above. Here, though, the figures are for the most common cause of death, coronary heart disease. The ratio of death rates for the 'worst health' decile compared to the 'best health' decile of areas rose from 1.89 between 1981-85 to 2.35 10 years later. People living in the 'worst health' 10% of Britain are now more than twice as likely to die as a result of coronary heart disease before the age of 65 than are people living in the 'best health' 10% of areas. Analysis of population deciles shows that 60% of the population have experienced declining relative as well as absolute mortality from coronary heart disease, but the 20% with the worst health have experienced increasing mortality from this cause in relative terms.

Table 4.7: **Change in mortality rates by age in the extreme areas of Britain (1981-85 to 1991-95) (% change)**

				Age		
Rank	**Name**	**0**	**1 to 4**	**5 to 14**	**15-44**	**45-64**
'Worst health' less 'best health' areas		*+18*	*+35*	*+17*	*+24*	*+16*
1	Glasgow Shettleston	-20	-15	-63	28	-6
2	Glasgow Springburn	-45	-27	-3	8	-7
3	Glasgow Maryhill	-36	0	-9	12	-10
4	Glasgow Pollok	-37	-71	1	11	-9
5	Glasgow Anniesland	-2	37	-17	4	-9
6	Glasgow Baillieston	-19	38	-2	-9	-9
7	Manchester Central	-38	-10	-54	8	-22
8	Glasgow Govan	-14	36	-20	7	-11
9	Liverpool Riverside	-44	-48	16	-15	-12
10	Manchester Blackley	-41	-15	-27	39	-18
11	Greenock and Inverclyde	-26	16	-77	-9	-15
12	Salford	-47	53	22	-7	-19
13	Tyne Bridge	-16	29	-62	12	-21
14	Glasgow Kelvin	-50	-2	65	-20	-18
15	Southwark North and Bermondsey	19	53	-33	44	-17
'Worst health' million		*-28*	*-4*	*-25*	*7*	*-14*
Rank	**Name**					
1	Wokingham	-18	21	-35	-14	-35
2	Woodspring	-64	-37	-64	-25	-31
3	Romsey	-49	-81	-10	-32	-33
4	Sheffield Hallam	-52	-24	-28	-33	-35
5	South Cambridgeshire	-49	-56	-27	-12	-28
6	Chesham and Amersham	-50	17	-43	-17	-28
7	South Norfolk	-60	-54	-34	-18	-32
8	West Chelmsford	-47	-61	-68	0	-37
9	South Suffolk	-57	-66	-45	-4	-41
10	Witney	-29	49	-24	-1	-33
11	Esher and Walton	-40	-43	-73	-8	-31
12	Northavon	-40	-41	-27	-26	-29
13	Buckingham	-41	-23	-57	-24	-39
'Best health' million		*-46*	*-39*	*-42*	*-17*	*-33*
Britain		**-38**	**-33**	**-26**	**-5**	**-28**

Note: Change figures for individual places are variable, but the aggregate trend is robust.
Source: Analysis by authors

Figure 4.7: **Absolute change in mortality rates of people aged 15-44 in the extreme areas of Britain (1981-85 to 1991-95)**

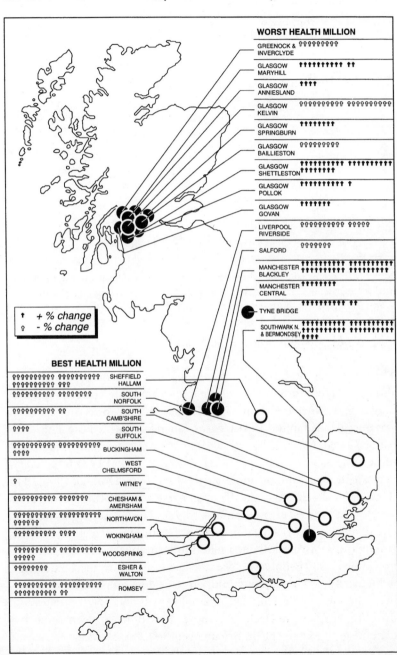

Source: Table 4.7

Table 4.8: Deaths under 65 from coronary heart disease (CHD) by
population deciles in Britain (1981-85 and 1991-95)

Decile	Number of CHD deaths < 65		SMR 1981-85	SMR 1991-95	% change in SMRs 1980s-90s
	1981-85	1991-95			
1	26,589	16,947	138.4	158.9	20.5
2	23,803	15,013	127.4	136.9	9.4
3	22,620	13,633	121.8	121.2	-0.6
4	19,924	12,747	110.8	112.3	1.5
5	18,187	11,547	100.2	97.0	-3.2
6	17,439	11,112	97.3	93.6	-3.7
7	15,479	9,977	88.0	84.3	-3.6
8	15,580	9,752	86.8	80.0	-6.8
9	14,409	9,068	82.5	76.4	-6.0
10	13,605	8,170	73.4	67.7	-5.7
Britain	187,635	117,966	103.1*	101.7*	-1.3

Note: SMRs for Britain are higher than 100 and rising as England and Wales rates are
used as the base for calculating these and as rates of CHD are high in Scotland.
Source: Analysis by authors; see Table 4.3

Inequalities between areas – morbidity

The polarisation in health is not only apparent in terms of mortality but
also in terms of morbidity. Limiting long-term illness (LLTI), a question
on which was included in the 1991 Census and is reported in Chapter 3,
was not included in the 1981 Census. Therefore, to see how illness rates
have changed over time by area, an alternative statistic must be used. The
most comparable Census question between 1981 and 1991 is the rate of
permanent illness among adults aged 16 and over (Dorling, 1995). This
was roughly 2% in Britain in 1981 rising to 4% by 1991. However, in the
'worst health' areas, it rose from 3% to 9%. This is over eight times the
rate of increase experienced in the 'best health' areas. In absolute terms,
among the 'worst health' one million in terms of their health, there are
now over 77,000 people who claim to be permanently sick, compared to
just under 18,000 in the 'best health' areas. Figures for permanent sickness
may sometimes reflect hidden unemployment and may not always be
disabling sickness; nevertheless, the polarisation between these two
extreme groups of people in Britain over the 1980s is striking.

Figure 4.8 maps the increases in the absolute numbers of people who
can no longer work in the extreme areas of Britain due to permanent

sickness. Note that it is the rates shown in Table 4.9 which are most strictly comparable, but here we show the absolute figures as these are more sobering. In the very worst off areas almost 4,000 additional adults are unable to work due to the increase in permanent sickness that occurred there during the 1980s and early 1990s. While this may not accurately measure disabling sickness, it has occurred at its greatest frequency in the areas in which we have also shown that there have been absolute increases in the mortality rates of young adults (Figure 4.7).

Table 4.9: **People with permanent sickness and unable to work, over age 15 in Britain (1981 and 1991)**

Rank	Name	Number in 1991	% in 1981	% in 1991	% change	Increase
	Ratio of 'worst health' to 'best health' areas	**4.4**	**2.7**	**4.5**	na	na
1	Glasgow Shettleston	5,663	4	12	7	3,370
2	Glasgow Springburn	5,764	4	11	7	3,452
3	Glasgow Maryhill	5,897	3	10	7	3,884
4	Glasgow Pollok	5,116	4	9	5	2,511
5	Glasgow Anniesland	5,085	4	9	5	2,627
6	Glasgow Baillieston	6,440	4	11	8	3,986
7	Manchester Central	6,452	4	9	5	3,412
8	Glasgow Govan	3,688	2	7	5	2,383
9	Liverpool Riverside	6,576	4	10	6	3,332
10	Manchester Blackley	5,440	3	8	5	2,888
11	Greenock and Inverclyde	4,098	3	8	5	2,349
12	Salford	5,153	4	8	4	2,399
13	Tyne Bridge	5,511	4	8	5	2,740
14	Glasgow Kelvin	3,015	2	6	4	1,849
15	Southwark North and Bermondsey	3,147	2	5	2	1,852
	'Worst health' million	*77,045*	*3*	*9*	*5*	*43,034*
Rank	**Name**					
1	Wokingham	931	1	1	0	486
2	Woodspring	1,642	2	2	0	484
3	Romsey	1,161	1	2	1	537
4	Sheffield Hallam	1,456	1	3	1	773
5	South Cambridgeshire	1,456	1	2	1	846
6	Chesham and Amersham	1,256	1	2	1	676
7	South Norfolk	1,743	2	2	1	647
8	West Chelmsford	1,215	1	2	1	633
9	South Suffolk	1,460	2	2	0	483
10	Witney	1,354	1	2	0	460
11	Esher and Walton	1,313	1	2	1	563
12	Northavon	1,598	2	2	0	482
13	Buckingham	1,094	2	2	0	236
	'Best health' million	*17,679*	*1*	*2*	*1*	*7,306*
Britain		1,795,647	2	4	2	926,923

Source: Analysis by authors of the 1981 and 1991 population Censuses

Figure 4.8: The numbers of people unable to work due to permanent sickness in the extreme areas of Britain (1981-91)

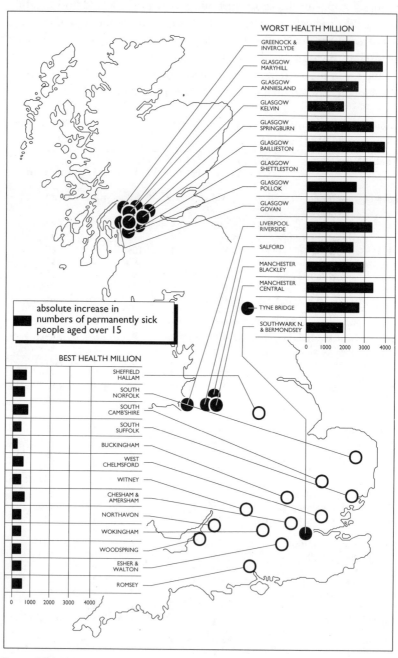

Source: Table 4.9

The widening employment gap

The increase (and geographical and social divergence) in the number of people unable to work because they are permanently sick is just one aspect of the changes in access to employment which have been partly responsible for the widening health gap. Although polarising rates of permanent sickness are clearly linked to widening inequalities in health, many major changes in employment may have contributed to the health gap widening rapidly in the 1980s and 1990s.

Changes in the world of work – non-employment

Over the past two decades in Britain, there have been radical shifts in the world of work. The number of people in employment has increased, especially the number of women working part-time. The total number in employment has risen from 23.9 million in 1986 to 25.9 million in 1997 (with most of the gain being in part-time and self-employment; Pullinger, 1998). However, this increase has not been evenly distributed. Instead, there has been an increase in 'work rich' households, where more than one person is in paid work. The number of people with second jobs had also increased to 1.3 million by 1997. This has been accompanied by an increase in 'work poor' households, with no member in paid employment. There has been a rise in the number of working-age families without anyone in work and this has contributed to a widening of the gap between the incomes of those in work and those not in work. As a result of these trends, between 1979 and 1995/96 in Britain there has been:

- an increase in the proportion of the population living in workless households from 7% to 18% of all working age people;
- a dramatic increase from 9% to 23% in the proportion of children without a working parent. Indeed, using a wider definition of worklessness, by 1995/96, 32% of children lived in families without a full-time worker (DSS, 1998a).

The polarisation of work is largely due to the rise in unemployment, and the concentration of unemployment in particular households. There has also been a rise in the economic inactivity of people on the edge of the labour market. The growth of dual earner households has exacerbated this polarisation, however, it is mainly the very low levels of welfare and unemployment benefit for those without work which affect ill-health. Not having work itself is not the root of the problem. In plain terms, very rich people who don't have to work don't appear to suffer from not working. There has also been a rise in single adult households and part of that rise is made up of an increasing number of households with only one parent present and of lone pensioner households (Table 4.10).

Table 4.10: Composition of households in Britain (as a % of all households) (1961-96)

	1961	1971	1981	1991	1995-96
One-person households over pensionable age	7	12	14	16	15
Lone parents with dependent children	2	3	5	6	7

Source: Adapted from Church and Whyman (1997)

These trends have been reported widely, but it is worth reiterating their impact in one simple summary. Gregg and Wadsworth (1996) refer to this "profound change in the distribution of work across households" as "more work for fewer households", they say:

> The number of households without a working member rose sharply in the recession of the early 1980s but nearly all of the subsequent recovery in employment occurred in households with one person already in work, leaving on balance many more multi-income households and twice as many workless households. By 1993, 14 per cent of individuals were resident in households with no work. Britain has become characterised by work-rich and work-poor families. (Gregg and Wadsworth, 1996, p 204)

People in the workforce – social class

Just as there are some minor problems in comparing the Censuses in terms of unemployment, comparisons by social class also require some care. The 1981 Census only provided counts of adults by social class who were economically active and so it is necessary to compare the class structure of the whole workforce rather than of just people in employment. More importantly, the Census authorities did not allocate any of the 920,000 people who were in the workforce but had never worked (mainly young adults) to a social class. They have been included in the 'other' category here and the effect of this is substantial. Nationally, the British workforce polarised in terms of social class over the 1980s.

The proportion of economically active people in social classes I and II rose, as did the proportion in the 'other' category, due entirely to the rise in adults who had either never worked or had not had employment in the last 10 years. The proportions in all other classes fell. If people who have never worked, but are unemployed (and are thus in the labour market) are excluded, then it appears that there is no class polarisation in Britain. This has been a common mistake of much Census-based social class analysis.

It is widely believed that the 'lower' social classes have shrunk in size but part of this shrinkage has been the growth in the numbers of people who cannot be assigned to a class because they have never worked. In reality, both ends of the social spectrum have grown over the last 20 years. There are now both more rich people and more poor people living in Britain.

Table 4.11 shows how the polarisation of people by social class (and 'classlessness' for the never employed 'other' category) was manifest geographically in the 'worst' and 'best' health areas of Britain. As we know from Table 4.5 above, the population aged under 65 in the 'worst health' areas fell, while those in the 'best health' areas rose. We need to take this into account as well as the changing proportions of people of working age in the workforce in each area (ie people working or available for work – the first column in Table 4.11). Having done that, we find that the proportion of the workforce in social classes I and II rose fastest in the 'worst health' areas but so did the proportion in the 'other' category. This is because, by 1991, over 10% of the economically active population of the 'worst health' areas had never worked. These areas saw a polarisation by class but changes in the overall social class composition were not highly correlated with changes in mortality in these places. Just as the traditional social class stratification does not work well for describing the living standards of many people in Britain today (see Chapter 2), it is a particularly poor indicator of how those living standards are changing. We include it here because it is widely used in other research and because it is still useful when attempts are made to take into account the large numbers of people who are unclassified by traditional classifications.

Figure 4.9 illustrates clearly how the rise in the numbers of people of working age who cannot be assigned a social class has been concentrated into the 'worst health' areas of Britain. Although the areas vary in the trends shown, in all the 'worst health' areas there are rapidly increasing numbers of adults who have never worked or not worked in the last 10 years.

Table 4.11: Change in social class of people in the workforce aged over 16 in the extreme areas of Britain (1981-91)

Rank Name		Workforce change	% change in social class share of workforce			
			I & II	III	IV & V	Other
'Worst health' less' best health' areas		**-40**	**+2**	**-2**	**-5**	**+5**
1	Glasgow Shettleston	-19	8	-3	-11	7
2	Glasgow Springburn	-30	6	-6	-7	6
3	Glasgow Maryhill	-18	11	-6	-11	5
4	Glasgow Pollok	-27	7	-7	-6	6
5	Glasgow Anniesland	-28	8	-6	-7	5
6	Glasgow Baillieston	-29	7	-3	-8	4
7	Manchester Central	-30	8	-6	-7	6
8	Glasgow Govan	-9	12	-10	-5	4
9	Liverpool Riverside	-35	7	-2	-14	9
10	Manchester Blackley	-20	5	-5	-4	5
11	Greenock and Inverclyde	-13	5	-6	-2	3
12	Salford	-27	8	-2	-8	3
13	Tyne Bridge	-15	3	-3	-7	7
14	Glasgow Kelvin	-8	12	-7	-8	3
15	Southwark North and Bermondsey	-3	15	-8	-12	5
'Worst health' million		-22	8	-5	-8	5
Rank Name						
1	Wokingham	51	8	-4	-4	0
2	Woodspring	13	4	-2	-2	0
3	Romsey	17	7	-5	-2	-1
4	Sheffield Hallam	2	8	-7	-2	1
5	South Cambridgeshire	14	7	-4	-2	0
6	Chesham and Amersham	9	6	-3	-2	0
7	South Norfolk	19	5	-4	-2	1
8	West Chelmsford	14	5	-3	-3	0
9	South Suffolk	20	5	-2	-4	1
10	Witney	24	7	-1	-5	-2
11	Esher and Walton	5	7	-6	-2	0
12	Northavon	25	2	-1	-1	-1
13	Buckingham	25	6	-1	-4	-1
'Best health' million		18	6	-3	-3	0
Britain		4	6	-4	-3	1

Note: Figures are from the 10% sample of the population Censuses. The % point change statistics sum to zero for each area or group of areas. Workforce change is change in the proportion of adults of working age in the workforce over this period. The % point changes are of changes in the distribution of social classes within this changing workforce.

Source: Analysis by authors of the 1981 and 1991 population Censuses

Figure 4.9: **Change in people of working age with no social class in the extreme areas of Britain (1981-91)**

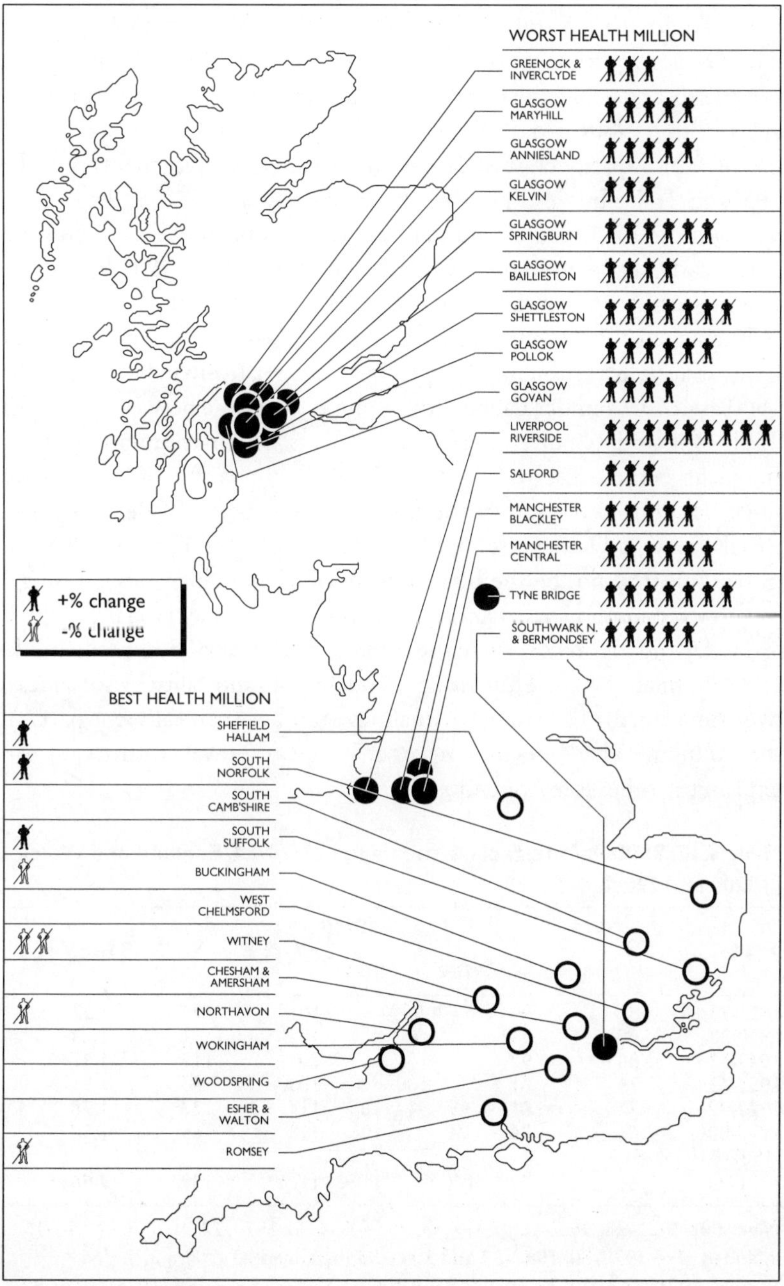

Source: Table 4.11

Historical polarisation of mortality by social class

Social class is based on occupation and while this may not be as inclusive as we would like, it is still the traditional way of looking at the health gap. The previous section showed how the social class of people in work is not the most useful explanation for rising mortality differences between areas in the 1980s and 1990s. However, historically it has been more useful. This is partly because Britain had near full employment from the 1950s to 1970s but also because the social class system was devised for use with the 1911 Census and so categorises people in ways which were particularly pertinent to the start of this century. Table 4.12 below shows that inequalities in mortality by social class were high in the 1920s, but only reached this extreme again in 1963 (following the first post-war Conservative government). Inequalities were relatively stable during the 1960s and 1970s under Labour rule – just as they were between areas (see Table 4.4 and Chapter 5 on the impacts of government policy). Inequalities then rose to very high levels in the early 1980s and have since continued to rise. In the table the ratio between death rates in social class V and I are presented. As the social class groups have changed in size this may not be the best measure of changes over time. Using a more robust method for quantifying inequality across social classes, which is not dependent on the size of the groups, yields similar findings (Pamuk, 1985; Najman, 1993). Thus rising inequalities in mortality by social class over time mirror the rising inequalities seen between different parts of the country. That does not necessarily mean, however, that one can explain the other (see Appendix C).

Table 4.12: SMRs by social class, men aged 15/20-64, England and Wales (1920s to 1990s)

Year	I	II	III		III	IV	V	Ratio V:I
			IIIN		IIIM			
1921-23	82	94		95		101	125	1.52
1930-32	90	94		97		102	111	1.23
1949-53	86	92		101		104	118	1.37
1959-63	76	81		100		103	143	1.91
1970-72	77	81	99		106	114	137	1.78
1979-80/ 1982-83	66	76	94		106	116	165	2.50
1991-93	66	72	100		117	116	189	2.86

Note: For 1921-23, 1930-32, 1949-53, 1959-63 and 1970-72 men aged 15-64 are included. For 1979-80/1982-83 and 1991-93 men aged 20-64 are included.
Sources: 1921-23, 1930-32, 1949-53 and 1959-63 from Thompson (1975); 1970-72 and 1979-80/1982-83 from Blaxter (1991); 1991-93 from Drever (1997)

Death rates

To understand the nature of this rise in inequalities in health by social class we need to consider who this is affecting most. This we can do by comparing mortality rates by class, by age group, over time. This comparison can only be made for men as women are often not classified under the social class schema (Smith and Harding, 1997). Table 4.13 shows that the ratio between the death rates of social class V and social class I has been getting steadily larger since the 1960s after some narrowing between the 1920s and 1950s. The ratios are greatest, however, for the youngest age groups: for men aged 25-34, those in social class V had death rates almost five times those in social class I by the early 1990s.

***Table 4.13:* Mean annual death rates (all causes) per 100,000 men by age and social class, England and Wales (1921-23, 1930-32, 1949-63, 1970-72, 1979-80 and 1982-83 and 1991-93)**

Age		Social class				
(years)	Year	I	II	IV	V	Ratio V:I
25-34	1921	261	376	420	498	1.9
	1931	288	283	360	374	1.3
	1951	147	112	172	224	1.5
	1961	82	81	119	202	2.5
	1971	65	73	114	197	3.0
	1981	54	62	106	204	3.8
	1991	39	57	96	187	4.8
35-44	1921	484	589	669	880	1.8
	1931	439	468	609	667	1.5
	1951	241	232	291	417	1.7
	1961	166	177	251	436	2.6
	1971	168	169	266	394	2.3
	1981	114	131	233	404	3.5
	1991	101	111	195	382	3.8
45-54	1921	985	1,090	1,173	1,507	1.5
	1931	984	1,021	1,158	1,302	1.3
	1951	792	706	725	1,041	1.3
	1961	535	545	734	1,119	2.1
	1971	506	564	818	1,069	2.1
	1981	398	462	728	1,099	2.8
	1991	306	314	545	916	3.0
55-64	1921	2,247	2,469	2,482	3,061	1.4
	1931	2,237	2,347	2,340	2,535	1.1
	1951	2,257	1,957	2,105	2,523	1.1
	1961	1,699	1,820	2,202	2,912	1.7
	1971	1,736	1,770	2,362	2,755	1.6
	1981	1,267	1,439	2,082	2,728	2.2
	1991	953	1,002	1,620	2,484	2.6

Source: Blane et al (1997)

Years of potential life lost by social class

There are methods of measuring inequalities in mortality other than by comparing SMRs. One of these is to measure the number of years of life which people do not live to experience because they died early. It has been claimed that it is important to consider these measures because SMRs "fail to register fully the extent to which deaths in manual social classes occur at younger ages, thus producing conservative estimates of the size of mortality differentials" (Blane and Drever, 1998). The calculation of years of potential life lost takes into account age at death as well as death itself.

Table 4.14 shows the number of years of potential life lost (due to early death) for every 1,000 of the population for men aged 20-64 in the various social classes. This includes all causes of death and has taken into account the different age structures of different social classes (social class I, for example, tends to be older, partly because of the years of education and training needed to qualify for many professions).

Table 4.14: Annual age-adjusted rate of years of potential life lost per 1,000 population (all causes of death), men, England and Wales (1970-93)

Social class	1970-72	1979-80, 1982-83	1991-93
I	48.7	36.5	28.0
II	51.9	42.2	31.6
IIIN	65.0	53.9	45.7
IIIM	66.0	58.0	50.5
IV	75.6	67.7	52.8
V	103.0	105.8	93.3
Ratio I:V	**2.1**	**2.9**	**3.3**

Source: Blane and Drever (1998)

The ratio of years of potential life lost between social classes V and I widened from 2.1 in 1970-72 to 2.9 in 1979-80 and 1982-83, and widened even further to 3.3 in 1991-93. This means that, for people assigned to social class V, there were over three times as many years of potential life lost than for those classed as social class I. Blane and Drever (1998) point out that much of this widening has been accounted for by deaths due to accidents and violence, which tend to occur in earlier adulthood than other causes of death, such as heart disease. Thus, measuring the growing polarisation of mortality by SMR and occupational class underestimates the extent of the problem not only because not everyone has a social class, but also because SMRs do not put great weight on the youngest deaths that occur disproportionately to the poorest in society.

Unemployment and widening inequalities in health

A significant area of government policy concerns the reduction of unemployment, but reducing unemployment will not necessarily, nor by itself, reduce inequalities in health. What matters most in terms of inequalities in health is to reduce long-term unemployment, not just the headline rate. In the government publication *Health inequalities* (1997), Bethune reports that mortality differences between the unemployed and employed are narrowing, by referring to the data presented in Table 4.15 (figures are only available for men).

Table 4.15: **Mortality rates of men of working ages by economic activity at the 1971 and 1981 Censuses (1971 and 1981 LS cohorts), England and Wales (1971-89)**

	Rates per 100,000 people	
Economic activity	**1971-79**	**1981-89**
Employed	302	227
Unemployed*	410	319
Death rate ratio	**1.36**	**1.41**

Note: *For both these time periods unemployment was defined as seeking work or waiting to take up a job in the week preceding the Census.
Source: Bethune (1997)

We have added the third row to the table which shows that while the absolute difference in mortality rates has decreased if you consider the ratio of the two rates at the two time periods you see that the level of inequality has in fact risen. The ratio between the death rates of these two groups has widened, from 1.36 to 1.41. Thus the unemployed are now proportionately more likely to die young than those in employment. This is despite the fact that they now constitute such a large group; as unemployment has grown and increasing numbers of young people are now among the ranks of the unemployed, their death rates might be expected to be 'watered down' as unemployment became more common. However, this has not occurred because to be unemployed at a time of mass unemployment can be worse (and likely to last longer) than is unemployment during times when work is more plentiful (Dorling,

1995). Table 4.16 shows the effect of long-term unemployment on health. Although the people unemployed at both times could have been working in between Census dates, they are obviously representative of the long-term, or frequently, unemployed in society.

Table 4.16: The effect of long-term unemployment on mortality, men aged 25-64, England and Wales (1981-92)

Economic activity			Mortality 1981-92	
1971 Census	1981 Census	Number in LS in 1981	Deaths	SMR
Employed	Employed	90,831	4,660	83
Employed	Unemployed	7,007	512	127
Unemployed	Employed	2,172	124	127
Unemployed	Unemployed	1,904	100	194
Total		101,104	5,396	

Source: Bethune (1997)

Table 4.16 shows that the SMR is highest for those unemployed at both the 1971 and 1981 Censuses and that this is associated with the highest risk of mortality. Even when unemployment rates are stable, the length of time that people experience unemployment tends to rise as unemployment is concentrated within particular groups and within areas. Thus the effect of unemployment on health is mediated by length of exposure to unemployment, not merely by the headline rate of unemployment. This can clearly be seen by the concentration of people who have never had a job in the 'worst health' areas of Britain (see Figure 4.9). In spring 1996, 28% of unemployed men in their 40s had been unemployed for three years or more (Church and Whyman, 1997).

Changing inequalities in the labour market

Measuring the changing rates of employment and unemployment in Britain is particularly difficult as the definitions of unemployment change so frequently. One robust method is to compare people's own description of their current employment status in the national Censuses. Table 4.17 shows how many men aged 16 to 64 were neither employed full-time nor part-time in both 1981 and 1991. Nationally, by this measure of underemployment, 3.4 million men were lacking work in 1981, rising to 4.2 million in 1991. This represents a rise of 4% nationally but an increase of 9% in the 'worst health' areas where 43% of all men of these ages are not employed (compared to only 17% in the 'best health' areas). As the table shows, the increase in underemployment was 2.6 times higher in the 'worst health' areas compared to the 'best health' areas. It is possible that this is partly caused by increased numbers of men in the 'worst health' areas becoming university students or starting their own businesses and retiring early. It is more likely, however, that it is men becoming unemployed, dropping out of the labour market altogether, or becoming permanently sick and leaving the area to find work in other places which has led to this very sharp rise.

The geography of the increase in men of working age lacking work is shown in Figure 4.10. The uniformity of 10% and 11% rises in most of the 'worst health' areas of Britain is striking, as is the very low increase seen in all the 'best health' areas. The biggest increase has been in Glasgow Springburn, where a majority of men of working age no longer work. The same is true for Liverpool Riverside – which saw the second largest increase in joblessness for men in the 1980s.

The changing geography of employment and unemployment is even more stark where women are concerned. It is a great pity that statistics on unemployment and class for women have not been as routinely analysed in detail using the Longitudinal Study as they have been for men. Instead, Table 4.18 uses the national Census. This shows that between 1981 and 1991 there was a 6% national increase in the proportion of women aged between 16 and 64 in employment (which rose to 59% by 1991). In the working age group (16-59) this rise may be even steeper; however, the same age groups for men and women have been used for simplicity and so that these figures are comparable to the statistics for mortality ratios presented here. Despite this overall rise in women's employment, over the 1980s their employment rate actually fell by 4% in the 'worst health' areas while rising by 10% in the 'best health' areas. In 1981, women in the two groups of areas had practically the same chances of being in employment (just over 50%). By 1991, women in the 'worst health' areas were 40% more likely not to be in employment than those in the 'best health' areas. The rise in the proportion of women working in Britain has been highly geographically selective. The majority of women aged 16-64 in the 'worst health' areas of the country now do not work. This was not the case 10 years earlier when the majority did work.

Table 4.17: **Lack of work for men aged 16-64 in the extreme areas of Britain (1981-91)**

Rank	Name	Change %	No in 1981	% in 1981	No in 1991	% in 1991
	Ratio of 'worst health' to 'best health' areas	*n/a*	**2.9**	**2.4**	**2.4**	**2.6**
1	Glasgow Shettleston	11	7,571	37	9,265	49
2	Glasgow Springburn	16	8,821	35	10,081	51
3	Glasgow Maryhill	10	9,109	36	10,876	46
4	Glasgow Pollok	10	8,393	32	8,791	41
5	Glasgow Anniesland	10	8,095	33	8,231	43
6	Glasgow Baillieston	8	10,087	37	9,797	44
7	Manchester Central	10	14,592	40	14,690	50
8	Glasgow Govan	7	5,935	28	7,310	35
9	Liverpool Riverside	11	14,600	42	14,272	53
10	Manchester Blackley	10	8,765	29	10,441	39
11	Greenock and Inverclyde	9	6,098	27	7,199	36
12	Salford	8	9,589	32	9,779	40
13	Tyne Bridge	10	10,617	35	12,172	45
14	Glasgow Kelvin	7	5,890	31	7,464	38
15	Southwark North and Bermondsey	10	5,892	24	9,323	34
	'Worst health' million	*9*	*134,054*	*34*	*149,691*	*43*
Rank	**Name**					
1	Wokingham	2	2,580	12	4,342	14
2	Woodspring	3	3,825	15	5,113	18
3	Romsey	3	3,642	15	4,846	18
4	Sheffield Hallam	5	4,353	20	5,300	24
5	South Cambridgeshire	2	3,605	14	4,684	16
6	Chesham and Amersham	3	4,028	14	4,977	17
7	South Norfolk	2	3,747	14	4,817	16
8	West Chelmsford	4	3,310	11	4,853	15
9	South Suffolk	3	3,301	14	4,453	17
10	Witney	1	3,579	13	4,510	14
11	Esher and Walton	3	4,119	14	5,171	17
12	Northavon	2	3,927	14	5,324	16
13	Buckingham	3	2,927	13	4,291	16
	'Best health' million	*3*	*46,943*	*14*	*62,681*	*17*
Britain		**4**	**3,370,578**	**20**	**4,249,389**	**24**

Source: Analysis by authors of the 1981 and 1991 population Censuses

Figure 4.10: **Change in lack of work – men in the extreme areas of Britain (1981-91)**

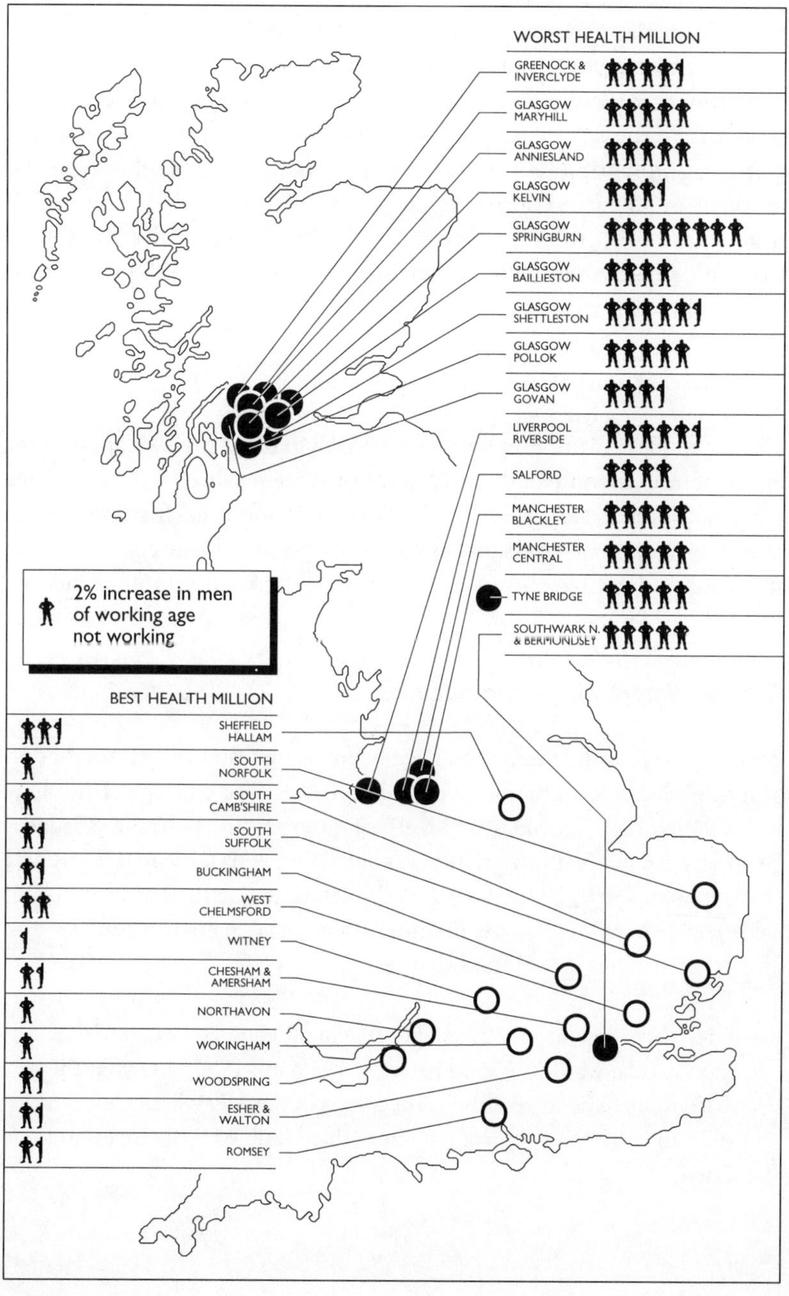

Source: Table 4.17

The extreme nature of the polarisation of women's work by area is made visual in Figure 4.11. In all but two of the constituencies in the 'worst health' areas of Britain the proportion of women not in work rose. Conversely, in every one of the 'best health' constituencies the proportion of women not in work fell by at least 5% and at most 14%. Thus the increase in women working is concentrated in the 'best health' areas where the largest numbers of men are also working. Here is the spatial manifestation of the increase in two-earner households in the south of England in contrast to the increase in no-earner households largely in the north and Scotland. It is the changing distribution of women's employment which explains much of the overall polarisation of households' fortunes.

The widening income gap

Changing patterns of employment are only part of the explanation for the widening income and wealth gaps in Britain which we claim drive growing inequalities in health. To look at household fortunes in the round, however, we need to consider changes in all sources of income and wealth. First we consider changes in those without either income or wealth – the poor.

Poverty – international comparisons

Poverty and income inequality have been rising faster in Britain than in other developed countries since the late 1970s. For example, Bradshaw and Chen (1997) looked at levels of poverty in Australia, Canada, Germany, Israel, the Netherlands, Norway, Sweden, Taiwan, the UK and USA at circa 1979, 1985 and 1990. Poverty was defined as households having below 50% average income after social security benefits and direct taxes. They concluded that:

> There has been an increase in poverty in all countries except Israel and Canada over this period between 1979 and 1990 but by far the sharpest increase in poverty has occurred in the UK where between 1979 and 1990 the poverty rate more than doubled. (Bradshaw and Chen, 1997, p 17)

Table 4.18: **Lack of work for women aged 16-64 in the extreme areas of Britain (1981-91)**

Rank	Name	Change %	No in 1981	% in 1981	No in 1991	% in 1991
	Ratio of 'worst health' to 'best health' areas	*n/a*	*1.3*	*1.0*	*1.4*	*1.4*
1	Glasgow Shettleston	6	10,349	51	10,963	57
2	Glasgow Springburn	8	12,628	48	12,673	57
3	Glasgow Maryhill	4	12,511	49	13,701	53
4	Glasgow Pollok	5	13,061	47	12,361	52
5	Glasgow Anniesland	5	12,437	46	11,400	51
6	Glasgow Baillieston	4	15,307	53	14,223	57
7	Manchester Central	7	17,419	51	17,609	59
8	Glasgow Govan	1	10,234	46	10,471	47
9	Liverpool Riverside	6	18,155	53	16,446	59
10	Manchester Blackley	6	13,205	45	14,088	51
11	Greenock and Inverclyde	-3	11,217	49	9,813	46
12	Salford	2	14,014	48	12,126	49
13	Tyne Bridge	2	14,814	51	14,160	53
14	Glasgow Kelvin	0	7,659	40	7,722	41
15	Southwark North and Bermondsey	7	9,868	40	13,342	46
	'Worst health' million	*4*	*192,878*	*48*	*191,098*	*52*
Rank	**Name**					
1	Wokingham	-11	9,200	44	9,851	33
2	Woodspring	-11	11,891	47	10,172	36
3	Romsey	-11	11,653	48	9,865	37
4	Sheffield Hallam	-6	10,116	45	8,575	39
5	South Cambridgeshire	-10	11,732	45	10,058	35
6	Chesham and Amersham	-8	13,415	46	11,169	38
7	South Norfolk	-11	13,127	49	11,673	38
8	West Chelmsford	-7	12,014	43	11,152	36
9	South Suffolk	-10	11,178	49	10,258	39
10	Witney	-12	11,960	46	10,303	34
11	Esher and Walton	-6	13,781	46	12,479	40
12	Northavon	-14	13,508	48	11,164	34
13	Buckingham	-10	10,205	47	9,402	37
	'Best health' million	*-10*	*153,780*	*46*	*136,121*	*37*
Britain		**-6**	**7,886,260**	**47**	**7,284,503**	**41**

Source: Analysis by authors of the 1981 and 1991 population Censuses

Figure 4.11: **Change in lack of work – women in the extreme areas of Britain (1981-91)**

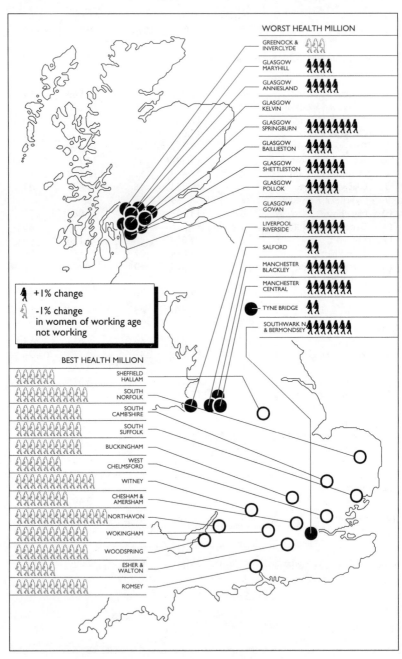

Source: Table 4.18

Other researchers have found that income inequality – the unequal distribution of income in the population – increased faster in Britain between 1967-92 than in comparable countries. Table 4.19 shows how the UK compares to other countries.

Table 4.19: Increases in income inequality, international comparisons (1967-92)

Increase	Country
More than 30%	UK
16-29%	USA, Sweden
10-15%	Australia, Denmark
5-10%	Norway, Netherlands, Belgium
Around 0%	Spain, France, Finland, Canada, Germany
Decreases	Italy

Source: Adapted by Lynch and Kaplan (1997) from Smeeding and Gottschalk (1996)

Over the same period (1967-92), the child poverty rate has also increased at a faster rate in Britain than in other comparable countries, many of which saw a reduction in this rate (Smeeding and Gottschalk, 1996).

The rapid growth of inequality and poverty in Britain can be clearly seen from official statistics on the percentage of the population living in households with incomes of less than half the average, after allowing for differences in housing costs. This is the poverty/income inequality measure that is currently favoured by both the British government and the European Statistical Office (Eurostat). Figure 4.12 shows that, during the 1960s, the amount of income inequality in Britain remained fairly constant with around 11% of the population living on incomes below half of the average. The recession and stagflation of the early 1970s caused the numbers living on less than half average incomes to rise to a peak of just over 13% in 1972. The relatively progressive government social and economic policies of the mid-1970s resulted in this measure of poverty falling rapidly to a low of under 8% of the population in 1977/78. The 1979 election victory of the Conservative Party under Mrs Thatcher's leadership reversed social and economic policies designed to promote equity and caused a rapid growth in poverty and inequality which increased throughout the 1980s and early 1990s. By 1995/96 almost a quarter (24%) of the British population was living on incomes that were below half the national average income.

Similarly, studies that examine poverty in terms of both low income and low standard of living have shown that poverty (using the *Breadline Britain* index) increased by almost 50% between 1983 and 1990. In 1983, 14% of households (approximately 7.5 million people) were living in poverty and, by 1990, 20% of households (approximately 11 million people) were living in poverty (Gordon and Pantazis, 1997). We mapped the locations of these households in Figure 2.3 and discussed the statistics for the 1990s in detail in Chapter 2.

Figure 4.12: **Percentage of the population with below half average incomes after housing costs (1961-95)**

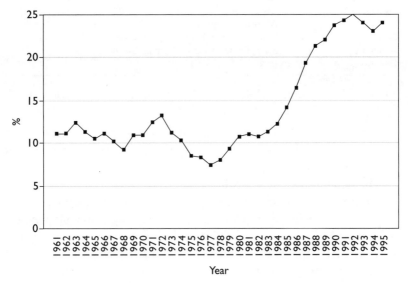

Year

Source: HBAI volumes (DSS, 1998a); Goodman and Webb (1995); Hills (1998)

The latest available figures from Eurostat for 1994 show that Britain now has more poor people than any other country in Europe. Table 4.20 shows the numbers and proportions of the populations of 14 European countries living on incomes below half of the average in their countries after allowing for differences in the purchasing power of the different currencies. In 1994, Britain is estimated by Eurostat to have almost 13.5 million people (23% of the population) living on incomes of less than 50% of the average. Poverty and income inequality using this definition is 23% in the UK. Only Portugal and Ireland have a greater proportion of their populations living in poverty.

Table 4.20: **Number and % of the population living on incomes below half of the average in 14 European countries (1994)**

Country	Number of people below 50% of average income	% of the population below 50% of average income
United Kingdom	11,427,766	20
Germany	11,328,673	14
Italy	9,322,853	17
France	7,949,907	14
Spain	7,196,406	19
Portugal	2,424,533	25
Greece	2,041,923	20
Belgium	1,474,158	15
Netherlands	1,275,048	8
Austria	1,108,082	14
Ireland	837,490	23
Denmark	386,015	7
Finland	192,153	4
Luxembourg	56,734	14

Source: Analysis by authors of unpublished data from the 1994 European Household Community Panel Survey (Eurostat, 1994)

Rising poverty in Britain

In Britain the income gap between the worst off and the best off has been widening over the past 20 years. Table 4.21 shows that, after housing costs, the richest 10% of the population have 27% of total income, whereas the poorest 10% have only 2.2% of total income in 1994/95. This compares to 21% and 4%, respectively, in 1979. Looking at the extremes, Britain is a country where, in 1996, the richest 50 people had income and wealth totalling over £34 billion (*The Sunday Times*, 14 April 1996); this is far in excess of the wealth and incomes of the 'poorest' 5.5 million.

Between 1951 and 1995, Gross Domestic Product (GDP) grew by an average of 2.4% per year and this is reflected in a growth in real income. Between 1961 and 1994, average real household disposable income (with the effects of inflation removed and net of taxes on income, National Insurance Contributions and local taxes) rose by 72%. However, this growth has not been evenly spread through the population. The proportion of households on low incomes (below half the national average) has risen, from one in ten in 1961 to one in five in 1990, although there was a slight improvement between 1992 and 1994, this proportion has risen again in recent years. As Church and Whyman note:

An important factor underlying these trends has been the widening of the earnings distribution. For men working full time the gap between the ten per cent with highest earnings and the ten per cent with lowest earnings was £203 per week in 1971. By 1995 this gap had increased to £419 per week. Both these figures are adjusted for inflation and based on April 1995 prices. For women, the gap grew from £122 to £290 per week over the same period. (Church and Whyman, 1997, p 39)

Table 4.21: **Distribution of income:** *Households Below Average Income* **series, Britain (1979 to 1994/95)**

Year	Poorest	2	3	4	5	6	7	8	9	Richest
	Share of successive tenths of individuals by equivalised disposable income (or who gets what share of income)									
Before housing costs										
1979	4.3	5.7	6.6	7.6	8.5	9.5	10.7	12.2	14.2	20.6
1981	4.0	5.6	6.5	7.4	8.4	9.5	10.7	12.2	14.5	21.1
1987	3.6	5.0	5.9	6.9	8.0	9.1	10.4	12.2	14.9	24.2
1990/91	2.9	4.5	6.0	6.0	8.0	9.0	11.0	12.0	15.0	26.0
1992/93	2.9	4.6	6.0	6.0	8.0	9.0	10.0	13.0	15.0	26.0
1994/95	3.2	4.7	6.0	6.0	8.0	9.0	10.0	12.0	15.0	26.0
After housing costs										
1979	4.0	5.6	6.6	7.5	8.5	9.5	10.8	12.3	14.3	20.9
1981	3.7	5.4	6.3	7.3	8.3	9.5	10.7	12.3	14.7	21.8
1987	2.9	4.6	5.6	6.7	7.6	9.1	10.6	12.3	15.1	25.0
1990/91	2.1	4.1	5.0	7.0	7.0	10.0	10.0	12.0	16.0	27.0
1992/93	1.9	4.1	5.0	6.0	8.0	9.0	10.0	13.0	15.0	28.0
1994/95	2.2	4.1	6.0	6.0	8.0	9.0	10.0	12.0	16.0	27.0

Note: Rows sum to 100%.
Source: Hills (1998)

This disparity can also be seen if we look at the average earnings of particular occupations. Figure 4.13 shows real gross weekly earnings adjusted for one time point (1997) and reveals that between 1981 and 1997 a cleaner (in occupational social class V) remained at the same level of approximately £200 per week. Medical practitioners, however (occupational social class I), have had a real increase in average earnings, from £600 to over £800 per week.

Figure 4.13: **Real gross weekly earnings*: by selected occupation†, Britain (1981-97)**

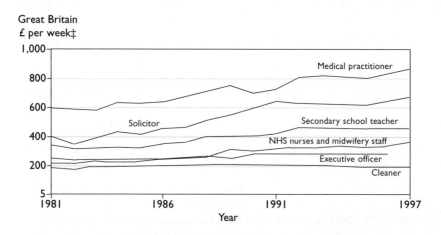

Great Britain
£ per week‡

Notes: * At April each year. Adjusted to April 1997 prices using the retail prices index. Full-time employees on adult rates whose pay was not affected for the survey period by absence. Before 1983 average earnings for men aged 21 and over and women aged 18 and over only.
† The definitions of some of the occupations shown experienced minor changes when the Standard Occupational Classification was introduced in 1990.
‡ Mid-point of the national pay scale, excluding local allowances.
Source: Pullinger (1998)

We can also consider changes in the income distribution for different types of households by looking at the 'top' and 'bottom' 10% of the population. Table 4.22 shows the changes in annual incomes of the poorest and richest 10% of families between 1979 and 1995/96. The poorest 10% of single adult households received, on average, £208 per year less in 1995/96 than they did in 1979 – they were absolutely poorer in real terms. By comparison, the richest 10% of single adult households were £6,968 richer in 1995/96 than in 1979. The situation was even more unequal for large families with three children where the poorest 10% were on average £625 poorer in 1995/96 compared with 1979 and the richest 10% were over £21,000 richer.

Table 4.22: **Change in annual incomes of the richest and poorest 10% of different types of families in Britain between 1979 and 1995/96 (in April 1998 prices)**

Family type	Poorest 10%	Richest 10%
Single adult	-£208	+£6,968
Couple with no children	-£364	+ £12,688
Couple with three children aged 3, 8 and 11	-£625	+ £21,164

Source: DSS (1998a)

This table indicates that, despite the overall picture of an increase in poverty in Britain between 1979 and 1995/96, some family types may have suffered even more than others.

Table 4.23: **Percentage of individuals below average percentiles of the income distribution, analysed by family type, after housing costs, including self-employed, Britain (1979 and 1995/96)**

	Bottom 10% of income distribution		Total population	
	1979	1995/96	1979	1995/96
Pensioner couple	20	3	9	9
Single pensioner	11	4	8	8
Couple with children	41	42	47	37
Couple without children	9	11	18	21
Single with children	9	17	4	8
Single without children	10	23	14	17

Source: Family Expenditure Survey, reported in DSS (1998a)

Table 4.23 shows the change in the percentage of individuals living in families in the bottom 10% of the income distribution in Britain between 1979 and 1995/96. It shows that pensioners have fared relatively better than younger families without children and lone-parent families. In 1979, 20% of individuals in the bottom 10% of the income distribution in Britain were living in pensioner couple families. However, by 1995/96 the proportion of individuals who were living in pensioner couples in the bottom 10% of the income distribution had fallen to just 3%. Conversely, 10% of individuals in 1979 in the bottom decile of the income distribution were young single people. However, by 1995/96 this had more than doubled to 23%. These changes can only partially be explained by the growth in single-person households over the 1980s and 1990s. The main reason for these relative changes in fortune of different family types is due to a range of government policies and socio-economic changes that have resulted in the impoverishment of many young single people, adolescents and children. For example, the series of social security changes during the 1980s which reduced the Income Support scale rates for people under 25 and made all under-18-year-olds ineligible for benefits resulted in severe hardship being experienced by many young people who could not find jobs. It also resulted in teenagers, with no other means of financial support, being forced to beg on the streets of all the major cities in Britain for the first time since the creation of the welfare state.

The widening wealth gap

We cannot state more clearly that it is this growth in inequalities in income and the consequent rise in poverty which most clearly underlies the widening of the health divide in Britain. Whether considering the processes that drive this change or the historical, spatial and social mirroring of income inequality and inequalities in health, the conclusion is the same. Most young deaths are due directly or indirectly to poverty and rising poverty leads to increasing inequalities in health. The relationships seen with social class and long-term unemployment are mostly reflections of this central cause.

Wealth in monetary terms

While income is a current measure of a person's economic position, wealth is a much better indicator of their economic position in the long term, as wealth is accumulated through the life-course. The inequality in wealth distribution has a similar pattern to that for income inequality (Hills, 1998) – wealth inequality fell at times before the 1980s but, since then, has changed little:

> The latest estimates give as large a share to the top 10 per cent in 1994 as in any other year since the official Inland Revenue series on this basis starts in 1976, and as great a share to the top 1 per cent as in any year since 1983. (Hills, 1998, p 18)

The distribution of wealth in the UK is markedly unequal. The most wealthy 1% of adults have consistently owned around 20% of the total marketable wealth over the past 20 years, as Figure 4.14 shows (Pullinger, 1998). Whether we consider the wealthiest 1%, 5%, 10%, 25% or the wealthiest 50%, the structure of wealth ownership has been stable over the past three decades.

Figure 4.14: The distribution of wealth in the UK, adults over 18 (1976-94)

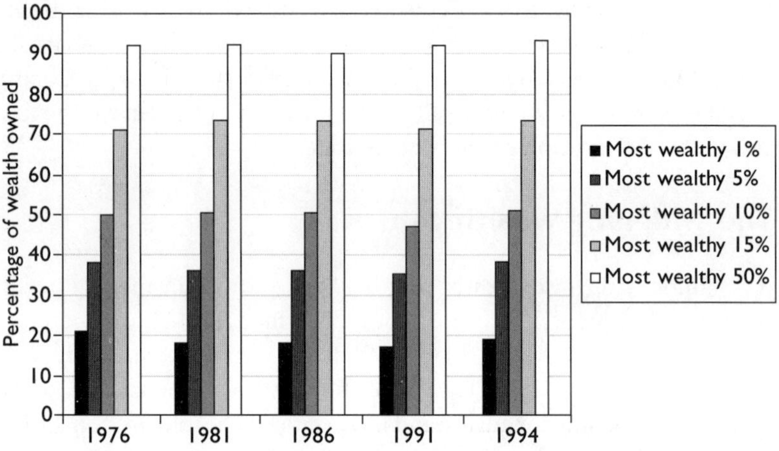

Source: Pullinger (1998)

The statistics presented in Figure 4.14 include wealth in the form of housing. Half of all marketable wealth in Britain is now held in the form of housing and thus it is important to consider housing wealth and the way in which housing is owned – tenure – in relation to rising inequalities in health.

Housing tenure

When considering advantage or disadvantage in terms of housing it is traditional to look at the tenure categories of home ownership, renting from a private landlord and renting from a social landlord (which includes council housing, and those renting from housing associations and Scottish Homes). Home ownership in Britain increased from 57% in 1981 to 68% in 1991 (Dorling, 1995). Other indicators of wealth rose similarly, the proportion of households with central heating increased from 37% in 1972 to 83% in 1992 and the proportion of households with more than one car increased from 9% in 1972 to 24% in 1992 (Wadsworth, 1996). However, the number of households in insecure housing tenures has also risen, reflected in increases in the number of mortgage repossessions and households in temporary accommodation – the number of which rose from over 10,000 in 1982 to over 67,000 in 1992 (Wadsworth, 1996). The number of households applying to local authorities as homeless and the number of single homeless has also risen (Victor, 1997).

Both owner-occupation and car ownership are reflections of wealth and hence of the likelihood of a person not living in poverty. Consequently we see from Table 4.24 that the relative mortality rates of people who are not owner-occupiers has risen between the 1970s and 1980s. This was a reflection of the polarisation of income and wealth among these tenure groups. A similar story can be seen in terms of access to cars.

Table 4.24: **Direct age-standardised rate ratios for deaths under 65 by housing tenure and car access: England and Wales, 1971 and 1981 Census cohorts (LS data)**

	Men		Women	
	1971-81	1981-89	1971-81	1981-89
Owner-occupiers	1	1	1	1
Private renters	1.32	1.38	1.32	1.38
Local authority tenants	1.35	1.62	1.42	1.44
1+cars	1	1	1	1
No cars	1.44	1.57	1.40	1.56

Source: Adapted from Filakti and Fox (1995)

Shelter (1998) estimates that 103,000 households in priority need were accepted for rehousing in 1997, with nearly 60% of them including children. This means that over 70,000 children faced the trauma of homelessness in that year. In addition, over 10,000 women faced losing their homes – and this includes only the official homeless. Shelter estimated that at the end of March 1998 over 32,000 children were living in temporary accommodation including hostels, Bed & Breakfast hotels and refuges. The detrimental effects of the experience of homelessness on children include emotional problems and behavioural difficulties. Difficulties also arise from moving schools (and thus housing influences education – see next section). A Shelter report in 1995 found that the introduction of school league tables meant that schools are often unwilling to spend time and resources on children with emotional and behavioural difficulties as it reflects badly on the performance of the school (Power et al, 1995). The upheaval of homelessness, which often means moving between areas, means that children lose contact with their friends, and in temporary housing they may not have access to safe play areas. Homelessness is yet another expression of poverty arising from inequality. It is also another example of a group who fall out of the traditional categories and hence are harder to measure – in this case a group without tenure.

Education and wealth

The advantages of wealth take many forms and one clear form is through access to education. The children of people living in wealthier neighbourhoods tend to have access to schools where their children are more likely to pass exams. If wealthy people do not have this access through the state they can purchase it from private schools. Access to universities is the most polarised of all forms of this kind of 'wealth'. As Table 2.6 showed, children living in the 'worst health' areas of Britain are many times less likely to go to university than are those living in the 'best health' areas. Wealth can be directly passed on as advantage through inheritance, but it is also passed on more subtly from parents to children through educational opportunities.

In Chapter 2, it was shown how there was little change in school exam results by area over the time period 1993-96 (Table 2.5). For a long-term perspective, we need to rely on the Census which only measures degree-level qualifications as an educational indicator. Table 4.25 shows the numbers and proportions of adults in work who had a degree-level qualification in 1981 and 1991 in the 'best' and 'worst' health areas that we have been following throughout this book. By 1991, only 16% of all adults in employment in the 'worst health' areas had degree-level qualifications but this was almost a doubling of the proportion in 1981 and represents a narrowing of the education divide between the two sets of areas. However, many of the 'worst health' areas are close to central city-based universities and hence their rates may be inflated by graduates from these universities working for a few years near to where they studied (and through postgraduate students working while continuing their studies).

Table 4.25: **Numbers and proportion of people in employment with degree level qualifications in Britain (1981 and 1991)**

Rank	Name	Adults in 1991 with a degree all (age 18+)	1981 % of all employed	1991 % of all employed	% increase 1981-91	Number increase
	Ratio of 'worst health' to *'best health' areas*	**44%**	**44%**	**65%**	**160%**	**40%**
1	Glasgow Shettleston	2,350	6	13	7	1,000
2	Glasgow Springburn	1,660	4	8	5	480
3	Glasgow Maryhill	4,390	7	18	11	2,320
4	Glasgow Pollok	2,440	5	10	5	630
5	Glasgow Anniesland	4,220	11	19	8	690
6	Glasgow Baillieston	1,730	5	7	2	120
7	Manchester Central	3,670	7	13	6	730
8	Glasgow Govan	6,410	17	25	8	1,760
9	Liverpool Riverside	4,610	11	19	8	400
10	Manchester Blackley	2,800	7	9	2	10
11	Greenock and Inverclyde	3,840	11	16	5	710
12	Salford	3,320	8	12	4	560
13	Tyne Bridge	2,600	7	9	3	230
14	Glasgow Kelvin	9,660	29	41	12	2,410
15	Southwark North and Bermondsey	6,030	5	18	13	4,390
	'Worst health' million	*5,9730*	*9*	*16*	*7*	*16,440*
Rank	**Name**					
1	Wokingham	13,280	22	29	6	6,410
2	Woodspring	8,910	20	21	1	1,670
3	Romsey	10,720	22	27	5	3,280
4	Sheffield Hallam	13,290	35	43	9	2,450
5	South Cambridgeshire	12,820	24	29	5	3,730
6	Chesham and Amersham	12,470	23	29	6	2,970
7	South Norfolk	7,700	13	17	4	2,750
8	West Chelmsford	10,270	19	21	3	2,380
9	South Suffolk	7,020	15	18	4	2,350
10	Witney	8,820	13	19	5	3,740
11	Esher and Walton	12,810	23	28	5	2,890
12	Northavon	9,790	17	19	3	3,120
13	Buckingham	9,280	19	24	5	3,390
	'Best health' million	*137,180*	*20*	*24*	*4*	*41,130*
Britain		**4,183,020**	**13**	**17**	**4**	**1,173,130**

Source: Analysis by authors of the 1981 and 1991 Censuses of population (10%)

Figure 4.15: Increase in numbers of people with university degrees in the extreme areas of Britain (1981-91)

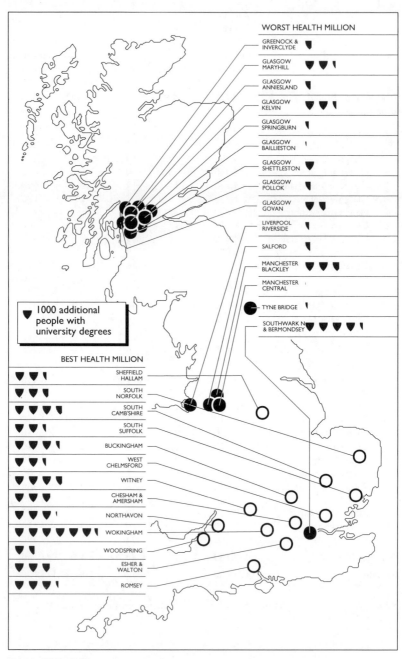

WORST HEALTH MILLION

GREENOCK & INVERCLYDE
GLASGOW MARYHILL
GLASGOW ANNIESLAND
GLASGOW KELVIN
GLASGOW SPRINGBURN
GLASGOW BAILLIESTON
GLASGOW SHETTLESTON
GLASGOW POLLOK
GLASGOW GOVAN
LIVERPOOL RIVERSIDE
SALFORD
MANCHESTER BLACKLEY
MANCHESTER CENTRAL
TYNE BRIDGE
SOUTHWARK N & BERMONDSEY

1000 additional people with university degrees

BEST HEALTH MILLION

SHEFFIELD HALLAM
SOUTH NORFOLK
SOUTH CAMB'SHIRE
SOUTH SUFFOLK
BUCKINGHAM
WEST CHELMSFORD
WITNEY
CHESHAM & AMERSHAM
NORTHAVON
WOKINGHAM
WOODSPRING
ESHER & WALTON
ROMSEY

Source: Table 4.25

The main superficial feature of education in Britain over the past two decades has been inclusion rather than exclusion (see Table 4.26). This is reflected by Table 4.25 above which shows a narrowing of the gap between areas in terms of educational qualifications. However, Figure 4.15 shows that although the education gap has narrowed in relative terms it is still widening in absolute terms as far as tertiary education is concerned. This is because fewer people are in work in the 'worst health' areas and thus a greater increase in having a degree for people in work is compatible with a smaller increase in the actual numbers of people with a degree in these areas. Other statistics show that education is becoming more widespread, if not necessarily more equitably delivered:

- Nursery education – among three- and four-year-olds in the UK, 58% attended school in 1996/97 compared with around 20% in 1970/71. However, it should be noted that there are marked differences in the availability of provision between local authorities (Pullinger, 1998) and of the quality of such nursery education.
- Higher education – the number enrolling on higher education courses between 1970/71 and 1995/96 – has more than trebled. Now one in three young people enter higher education:

> Young people are more likely than ever to either stay on at school to take A levels, attend vocational courses at colleges of further education or undertake government-supported training. Around three-quarters of those aged between 16 and 18 in England were in education and training at the end of 1996. (Pullinger, 1998, p 60)

Table 4.26: **Enrolments in further and higher education in the UK, for men and women, (1970/71 to 1995/96) (000s)**

	Men				Women			
	1970/71	1980/81	1990/91	1995/96	1970/71	1980/81	1990/91	1995/96
FE	1,007	851	987	1,100	725	820	1,247	1,496
HE	416	526	638	913	205	301	537	987

Note: FE = further education; HE = higher education
Source: Adapted from Pullinger (1998)

Class inequalities in education have been shown to have persisted throughout the post-war era, despite education policies which have been specifically designed to reduce inequalities in educational outcomes between social classes (Heath and Clifford, 1990). This may well be because policies such as the introduction of comprehensive education have prevented the situation becoming worse, rather than actually improving it. Some aspects of the current education system are clearly becoming more unequal. *The Times*, August 27, 1998 noted:

> A widening gap between the brightest teenagers and the growing number leaving school with no qualifications at all will be exposed today with the publication of this summer's GCSE results. More than 4 per cent of this summer's five million entries were awarded the coveted A* – by far the biggest proportion since the grade was introduced. The 54.7 per cent reaching the equivalent of the old 'O' level also represented a small improvement. However, more than 120,000 entries were unclassified and did not merit even the lowest of the eight grades. The number of failures rose by more than 50 per cent, only the second increase since the exam was introduced a decade ago.

Exclusion from school

While the total number of exclusions as a proportion of the total school population is small, this number has been rising sharply in recent years, as Figure 4.16 indicates. The groups of children who are more likely to be excluded are:

- children with special needs, who are six times more likely to be excluded;
- African–Caribbean children, who are six times more likely to be excluded;
- children in care, who are 10 times more likely to be excluded (Social Exclusion Unit, 1998).

Figure 4.16: Children permanently excluded from schools in England (1990-97)

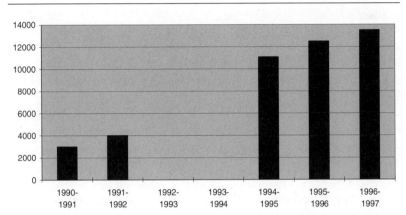

Note: Figures for the first two years were collected on a voluntary basis and so are almost certainly underestimates. There are no figures for 1992-93 and 1993-1994. The figure for 1996-97 is an estimate based on a sample of local education authorities. *Source:* Social Exclusion Unit (1998)

Growing income inequality has led to inequalities in wealth; these are reflected through inequalities in education and, at the extreme, are reflected through inequalities in the rare event of a child being excluded from school and the associated disadvantages that this entails. Much more common is general childhood poverty, experienced by 27% of households with children in Britain (Table 2.4). It is the changing distribution of childhood poverty that will have the greatest impact on inequalities in health in the future. How, though, has the distribution of childhood poverty been changing?

Childhood poverty

Limitations of the 1981 Census form constrain our ability to measure changes in childhood poverty over the last decade. The best comparable measure available is 'households with children with no adults in the workforce'. Table 4.27 shows that this rose from 4% of all households with children in 1981 to 10% in 1991 in Britain. However, the increase was much sharper in the 'worst health' areas, rising from 8% to 25% of all households with children. In the 'best health' areas, this measure rose from just 2% to only 4% of all households with children. The rate of increase in the 'worst health' areas was almost ten times that in the 'best health' areas. By 1991, almost 34,000 households with children in these areas had no adult in the workforce, compared with less than 6,000 in the 'best health' areas.

Figure 4.17 shows how there are now hundreds, and in most cases, thousands of additional households with children, but no adult in the workforce in the 'worst health' constituencies in Britain. These are households with children where there is no work but where no one is defined as unemployed, that is, where all the adults are either looking after the home, are permanently sick, early retired or are otherwise excluded from the workforce. These are mainly households with children which are both poor and are likely to remain poor and they have been concentrated most in the places which were poorest to begin with. There have also been small increases in the 'best health' constituencies – even here there are now more households with children where no one in the home is working – the polarisation of households into 'work rich' and 'work poor' has affected all parts of Britain. However, by far the greatest detrimental effects have been felt in the places which were poor to begin with and these influences will also be felt most by the children currently growing up in these places.

Inequalities in infant mortality

The widening gap in health by social class cannot only been seen in the mortality rates of adults. In the introduction to his last report as Chief Medical Officer, Sir Kenneth Calman highlights a number of overall improvements in health, including the fact that infant mortality has reached its lowest recorded rate, of 5.9 deaths per 1,000 live births (Calman, 1998). However, a closer inspection of these rates reveals that overall infant mortality rates have levelled off in the past four years and when these rates are considered by social class (of father) a different picture emerges. As Figure 4.18 below shows, there are growing differences between the death rates of babies with social class I fathers (professional occupations) and babies with social class V fathers (unskilled manual workers). Babies of unskilled manual workers are 2.2 times more likely to die than babies with fathers in professional occupations. For every 1,000 babies born whose father is social class V, eight babies died in their first year. In Table 2.2 we noted similar inequalities, but then when comparing communities where infant mortality rates are 2.0 times higher for those in the 'best health' areas compared to the 'worst health' areas.

Table 4.27: **Childhood poverty change: households with children with no adults in the workforce (1981 and 1991)**

Rank	Name	House-holds in 1991	1981 % of all house-holds	1991 % of all house-holds	% point increase 1981-91	Number increase
	Ratio of 'worst health' to 'best health' areas	**6.0**	**3.5**	**6.2**	**n/a**	**8.5**
1	Glasgow Shettleston	1,947	8	29	21	1,431
2	Glasgow Springburn	2,505	7	32	25	1,812
3	Glasgow Maryhill	2,518	8	29	21	1,769
4	Glasgow Pollok	2,039	6	23	16	1,360
5	Glasgow Anniesland	2,045	8	27	18	1,304
6	Glasgow Baillieston	2,737	8	27	19	1,736
7	Manchester Central	3,980	11	32	20	2,513
8	Glasgow Govan	1,337	5	19	14	955
9	Liverpool Riverside	2,982	11	29	18	1,559
10	Manchester Blackley	2,856	6	25	19	2,224
11	Greenock and Inverclyde	1,256	5	15	11	838
12	Salford	2,104	7	23	15	1,294
13	Tyne Bridge	2,527	8	24	16	1,589
14	Glasgow Kelvin	659	6	15	10	388
15	Southwark North and Bermondsey	2,484	10	25	15	1,678
	'Worst health' million	*33,976*	*8*	*25*	*18*	*22,450*
Rank	**Name**					
1	Wokingham	348	2	3	1	156
2	Woodspring	406	2	4	2	176
3	Romsey	420	3	4	1	153
4	Sheffield Hallam	347	3	5	2	145
5	South Cambridgeshire	354	2	3	1	115
6	Chesham and Amersham	437	2	4	2	257
7	South Norfolk	433	2	4	2	173
8	West Chelmsford	571	2	5	3	331
9	South Suffolk	514	2	5	3	274
10	Witney	432	2	4	2	187
11	Esher and Walton	629	3	5	3	355
12	Northavon	448	2	4	2	173
13	Buckingham	318	2	3	1	142
	'Best health' million	*5,657*	*2*	*4*	*2*	*2,637*
Britain		**652,395**	**4**	**10**	**6**	**382,293**

Source: Analysis by authors of the 1981 and 1991 population Censuses

Figure 4.17: **Change in households with children, living in poverty in the extreme areas of Britain (1981-91)**

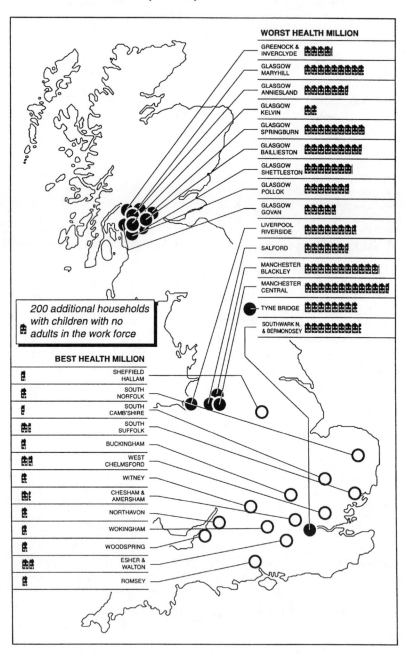

Source: Table 4.27

Figure 4.18: **Infant mortality by social class, England and Wales (1993-96)**

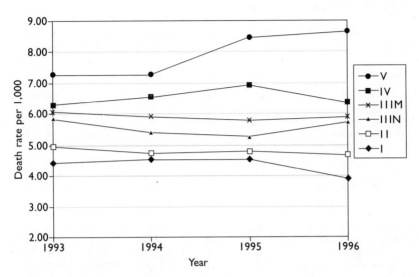

Source: ONS (1996, 1997, 1998b)

Rising numbers of avoidable deaths in Britain by age

If the infant mortality rate of babies born where the 'best health' million in Britain lived applied nationally, then some seven and a half thousand infants would not have died between 1991 and 1995 and a third of all infant deaths in Britain would be avoided. Ten years ago, the number was similar but the proportion was less than a quarter. Avoidable infant mortality in Britain has risen by 10 percentage points in 10 years. In the areas where the 'worst health' million now live, 364 babies died at the start of this decade who would not have died had rates in their areas been the same as the average for the 'best health' areas. This is exactly half of all the infant deaths that occurred in those areas. Ten years ago, fewer infant deaths were avoidable and the proportion was a third of all infant deaths in these areas. (Table 4.28 gives these figures for each area where the 'worst health' million people aged under 65 live.)

Table 4.28: **Avoidable infant mortality in the 'worst health' constituencies in Britain (1981-95)**

	Number 1981-85	% 1981-85	Number 1991-95	% 1991-95	% change
Britain	**7,644**	**22**	**7,567**	**32**	**10**
'Worst health' million	340	33	364	50	17
'Best health' million	0	0	0	0	0
Glasgow Shettleston	21	41	28	61	19
Glasgow Springburn	21	35	12	36	1
Glasgow Maryhill	15	29	15	41	12
Glasgow Pollok	30	40	20	49	9
Glasgow Anniesland	11	24	26	58	34
Glasgow Baillieston	13	19	21	46	27
Manchester Central	53	44	40	51	8
Glasgow Govan	10	19	21	50	30
Liverpool Riverside	26	29	13	31	3
Manchester Blackley	25	32	21	38	6
Greenock and Inverclyde	21	37	19	54	17
Salford	41	42	20	41	-1
Tyne Bridge	33	36	43	59	23
Glasgow Kelvin	8	26	3	21	-5
Southwark North and Bermondsey	13	23	63	65	42

Note: These are the number and proportion of deaths which would not have occurred, had mortality rates been the same as those for the 'best health' areas at each time period.
Source: Analysis by authors

A similar story is seen for deaths in childhood (Table 4.29) which, although rarer, are now just as polarised by area as infant mortality. This was not true of the early 1980s, but the degree of increase in polarisation over the subsequent decade was greater for childhood than infant mortality. Just under half the children who died in the 'worst health' areas in Britain at the start of this decade would not have died had they had the same chances as did children in the 'best health' areas. A decade before this, this proportion was a quarter. The proportion of deaths in childhood which are avoidable almost doubled during the 1980s. Note that the small numbers of deaths in some areas (in a few cases there are no deaths) reflect the relatively low numbers of children living in some of these areas. However, 144 children aged 1 to 14 died unnecessarily because of social inequalities in the 'worst health' areas. In Britain as a whole over one quarter of childhood deaths – those of 2,638 children – were attributable to social inequality.

Table 4.29: **Avoidable child mortality (aged 1 to 14) in the 'worst health' constituencies in Britain (1981-95)**

	Number 1981-85	% 1981 -85	Number 1991-95	% 1991 -95
Britain	**1,607**	**11**	**2,638**	**26**
'Worst health' million	*101*	*26*	*144*	*47*
'Best health' million	*0*	*0*	*0*	*0*
Glasgow Shettleston	9	42	4	33
Glasgow Springburn	7	27	8	49
Glasgow Maryhill	3	13	8	45
Glasgow Pollok	10	32	5	33
Glasgow Anniesland	2	10	7	45
Glasgow Baillieston	11	31	20	63
Manchester Central	22	44	15	48
Glasgow Govan	5	26	12	59
Liverpool Riverside	14	36	14	53
Manchester Blackley	11	33	14	49
Greenock and Inverclyde	0	n/a	0	n/a
Salford	2	6	18	60
Tyne Bridge	7	24	3	20
Glasgow Kelvin	0	0	1	25
Southwark North and Bermondsey	3	14	12	50

Source: Analysis by authors

Avoidable mortality in young adulthood (15-44) shows that an even greater proportion of deaths at these ages would be avoided were the rates in the 'worst health' areas the same as those in the 'best health' areas. A *majority* of all the young adults who died at the start of this decade, over two thousand people out of the population of a million aged under 65, would not have died had they enjoyed the life chances of their better off contemporaries (Table 4.30). Ten years ago, this proportion was smaller and accounted for over 600 fewer deaths. At some point during the late 1980s factors underlying health inequalities became the cause of the majority of deaths of young adults on the 'worst health' areas. In Britain as a whole, some eleven thousand young adults would not have had their deaths attributed to inequality in the early 1990s had inequalities in health not risen; almost thirty thousand young adults would be alive today if inequalities in health were eliminated. Instead, on average, 16 young adults die every day due to inequality and that number is steadily rising.

Table 4.30: **Avoidable young adult (15-44) mortality in the 'worst health' constituencies in Britain (1981-95)**

	Number 1981-85	% 1981 -85	Number 1991-95	% 1991 -95
Britain	17,532	17	28,572	28
'Worst health' million	*1,435*	*42*	*2,067*	*55*
'Best health' million	*0*	*0*	*0*	*0*
Glasgow Shettleston	110	54	196	70
Glasgow Springburn	149	55	176	66
Glasgow Maryhill	109	46	172	60
Glasgow Pollok	90	41	122	56
Glasgow Anniesland	97	45	117	56
Glasgow Baillieston	129	48	115	52
Manchester Central	125	41	193	54
Glasgow Govan	56	34	96	49
Liverpool Riverside	126	42	112	43
Manchester Blackley	79	35	196	61
Greenock and Inverclyde	94	46	86	51
Salford	96	40	104	46
Tyne Bridge	58	28	111	46
Glasgow Kelvin	54	35	49	33
Southwark North and Bermondsey	64	34	222	62

Source: Analysis by authors

Finally, in relative and absolute terms the most extensive divide can be seen for older adults aged 45-64 (Table 4.31). Nationally, a third of deaths in this age group (almost 30,000 deaths a year) would be avoided if the mortality rates in the 'best health' areas applied everywhere. In the areas where the 'worst health' million live, two thirds of deaths at these ages would be avoided. Two thirds of people who die before retirement age would not have died but for inequalities in health in Britain. If inequalities in health had not risen during the 1980s, if instead the improvement enjoyed by the 'best health' areas had been enjoyed by all, then one in 10 more people would have lived to reach retirement age from this age group. Instead, in today's Britain one adult aged over 44 dies every 20 minutes, both day and night, before reaching the age of 65, due to inequalities in health. The number is slightly less than a decade ago, not because of any fall in inequalities in health, but due to the overall improvement in health enjoyed by adults of this age. However, a far, far greater improvement could be achieved if inequalities in health were reduced, or even if their growth were simply halted. The fact that low mortality rates are possible in a minority of areas shows just what could be achieved, in terms of health in general, across all of Britain.

Table 4.31: **Avoidable older adult (45-64) mortality in the 'worst health' constituencies in Britain (1981-95)**

	Number 1981-85	% 1981 -85	Number 1991-95	% 1991 -95
Britain	**155,839**	**28**	**140,706**	**34**
'Worst health' million	*10,947*	*54*	*9,256*	*64*
'Best health' million	*0*	*0*	*0*	*0*
Glasgow Shettleston	822	60	769	72
Glasgow Springburn	881	59	787	70
Glasgow Maryhill	772	56	737	68
Glasgow Pollok	746	53	681	66
Glasgow Anniesland	676	51	577	64
Glasgow Baillieston	679	52	628	65
Manchester Central	1,080	58	723	64
Glasgow Govan	526	51	488	64
Liverpool Riverside	899	55	742	66
Manchester Blackley	763	52	619	61
Greenock and Inverclyde	554	50	508	61
Salford	817	54	610	62
Tyne Bridge	770	53	585	60
Glasgow Kelvin	540	55	416	63
Southwark North and Bermondsey	422	40	385	52

Source: Analysis by authors

Conclusion

We began this chapter by summarising some of the well-known facts about rising inequalities in many aspects of life in Britain. We then showed how inequalities in health have grown between different geographical communities; how this growth has followed growing inequalities in income; how it began between 1977 and 1981; how it was not always a feature of life in Britain; how inequalities had not increased in the 1960s and 1970s in both income and health; how these inequalities are now at their widest ever measured; how this affects the health of all age groups; how growing inequalities were also evident from statistics on illness; and how they are reflected by the underlying trends in income, poverty and wealth.

The core of this chapter examined what led to growing income inequality in Britain. We began by considering the polarisation of employment, unemployment and non-employment. We showed how the changing spectrum of social classes in Britain could not account for most of the growth in inequalities in health (see Appendix C). Instead we highlighted the importance of the rise in the number of people who have neither a job, nor the right to unemployment benefits, who are not assigned a social class, and most of whom have never worked. We showed also that rising unemployment on its own did not explain the growth in inequalities in health, rather that the rise in long-term and frequent unemployment was far more important. We concluded that most of what was thought to be explained through changes in employment, unemployment, occupation, tenure and car ownership were really reflections of the widening gap in the income distribution in Britain and the consequent rise in poverty that resulted from this.

Britain has experienced almost the fastest growth in income inequality in the developed world and has some of the highest levels of poverty seen within Europe. In Britain, more people are classified as poor by European Union statisticians in absolute numbers than in any other EU country. We showed how the nature of this poverty has changed over time, how it has grown in general but also become more concentrated in particular social groups. Most importantly the influence and incidence of poverty has grown most rapidly for children and young people and it is here that we have seen some of the greatest increases in inequalities in health. We then considered some of the possible mitigating effects of education and changes in educational provision over time, before concluding that the rapid rise in childhood and young people's experience of poverty far outweighed any advantages which may have occurred from wider participation in education.

We ended the chapter by documenting the exact numbers of babies, children and younger and older adults who would not have died during the first half of the 1990s in Britain had the health advantages of the 'best health' minority been enjoyed by the majority. We compared these numbers to the situation exactly 10 years previously and conclude the following: had inequalities in health not been allowed to rise during the 1980s as a direct consequence of rising inequalities in income, then thousands of people would not have died prematurely. Some 36,000 people a year died before age 65 in Britain due to inequalities in health. Most striking, the majority of both infants and people aged 15-44 who are dying would not be dying now were inequalities in health to be eliminated. This was not the case 10 years earlier. Inequalities in health for these two age groups now (and for all people aged under 65 in the near future) account for the majority of premature deaths in Britain. In the years to come, given current trends, inequalities in health and their determinants will be the underlying cause of the majority of mortality before age 65. In terms of health nothing is more important than eliminating these inequalities.

FIVE

Narrowing the gap – the policy debate

Summary

- The key policy that will reduce inequalities in health is the alleviation of poverty through the reduction of inequalities in income and wealth.

- There is widespread public support for poverty reduction in Britain and the government has pledged to eliminate childhood poverty by 2020.

- Poverty can be reduced by raising the standards of living of poor people through increasing their incomes 'in cash' or 'in kind'. The costs would be borne by the rich and would reduce inequalities overall – simultaneously reducing inequalities in health.

The purpose of this chapter is to examine the realistic policy options that would halt and then reduce the ever-widening health gap that has been documented in the four preceding chapters. The government White Paper on public health, *Saving lives: Our healthier nation*, published in July 1999, set out two key aims of the Labour government's health policy (DoH, 1999a). The first aim was to improve the health of the population as a whole by increasing the length of people's lives and the number of years spent free of illness. The second key aim was to improve the health of the worst off in society and to narrow the health gap (DoH, 1999a). In the White Paper, it is argued that these twin goals "are consistent with the health strategies being adopted by other countries of the United Kingdom" (DoH, 1999a). They are also consistent with the new programme of the World Health Organisation (Europe) for the 21st century, *Health 21* (WHO, 1999), and the European Community's developing strategy for public health (DoH, 1999a).

The first of the government's aims is the less challenging – average life expectancy in Britain has been rising since reliable data were first collected over 150 years ago (Charlton, 1997). Unless Britain suffers from an economic catastrophe, such as that which has befallen the former countries of the Soviet Union, it is likely that average life expectancy in Britain will continue to increase. It is the government's second aim of narrowing the health gap that will require major policy changes if it is to be realised. As the evidence presented in Chapter 4 showed, it has been the increases in poverty and income inequality that have preceded greater inequalities in health in Britain. The White Paper explicitly acknowledges this fact and states "the story of health inequality is clear: the poorer you are, the more likely you are to be ill and die younger" (DoH, 1999a).

Poverty and inequalities in health

The evidence that poverty and inequality in material well-being underlie inequalities in health is now overwhelming, as we have detailed in the earlier chapters of this book. Evidence which has accrued over the past two decades lends further support to the conclusion of the Black Committee on Inequalities in Health originally published in 1980 that:

> While the health care service can play a significant part in reducing inequalities in health, measures to reduce differences in material standards of living at work, in the home and in everyday social and community life are of even greater importance. (Townsend and Davidson, 1988, p 165)

The appropriate policies are those which recognise this fundamental fact and address themselves to the alleviation of poverty and the reduction of inequality, particularly as they influence people's lives around the key transition points highlighted in Box 3.1 in Chapter 3.

Of crucial importance here is the need to ensure an adequate and fair start to life for all children. For the Black Committee, the primary policy recommendation to improve inequalities in health was, therefore, the creation of a comprehensive anti-poverty strategy and, in particular, that "the abolition of child poverty should be adopted as a national goal for the 1980s".

The causal relationship between poverty and ill-health is now proven beyond any reasonable doubt and this has been acknowledged and accepted by the world's leading authorities on health and social development. In his Beveridge Lecture on 18 March 1999, Tony Blair committed the government to "lifting 700,000 children out of poverty by the end of the Parliament" and "to end child poverty for ever" over the next 20 years (Blair, 1999). He argued that "We have made children our top priority because as the Chancellor memorably said in his Budget 'they are 20% of the population but they are 100% of the future'". While it is welcome that the Black Committee's recommendation of two decades earlier has been accepted, to end child poverty 'for ever' over the next 20 years will require a lot more than just soundbites and good intentions.

A short history of Labour's policies on inequalities in health

While in opposition during the 1990s, the Labour Party made a series of promises to the people of Britain. At the core of those promises was a commitment to increase equality and the living standards of the poor and at the heart of Labour's concerns were inequalities in health. Tony Blair clearly stated Labour's commitment:

> I believe in greater equality. If the next Labour Government has not raised the living standards of the poorest by the end of its time in office it will have failed. (Tony Blair, 1996, quoted in Howarth et al, 1998, p 9)

A new ministerial post was created and the first Minister of Public Health, Tessa Jowell, in her first major speech after the election, made clear the government's intentions by stating:

> ... setting our mission to tackle the inequalities that give rise to ill health ... we propose to set new goals for improving the overall health of the nation which recognise the impact of poverty, poor housing, unemployment and a polluted environment.... We will wage war on inequalities where children's health is determined by the accident of their birth. (Jowell and DoH, 1997a)

However, once the euphoria of winning the election had waned, the government's approach began to change. Subtly, slowly and almost imperceptibly, the priority of reducing inequalities in health dropped down the agenda. The government appeared to have decided to act slowly on the issue. New Labour ministers discovered other priorities, for example, Stephen Byers, the Minister for Trade and Industry, argued that:

> The reality is that wealth creation is now more important than wealth redistribution. (quoted in Jones, 1999)

The need to maintain, for the first two years of government, the general fiscal framework of the previous government was seen as more important than extra government spending to reduce inequality and poverty. With little extra money for implementing concrete policies to reduce inequalities in health during the first two years, strategies for delay became essential to maintain credibility.

The new Labour government's flagship policy of Health Action Zones as a primary method for reducing inequalities in health was announced in a speech by Frank Dobson to the NHS Confederation on 25 June 1997, only one month after Labour's General Election victory. However, despite the early announcement, funding for the Health Action Zones (HAZ) was extremely limited during the first two years of government. The complex and lengthy bidding process meant that the first 11 were not set up in England until April 1998. The 11 successful HAZ were Bradford, the East End of London, Lambeth Southwark and Lewisham, Luton, Manchester Salford and Trafford, North Cumbria, Northumberland, Plymouth, Sandwell, the South Yorkshire Coalfield Communities and Tyne and Wear. However, between them, they only received extra resources amounting to £4m in 1998/99 to jointly spend with local authorities and other participating agencies.

A major Independent Inquiry into Inequalities in Health, chaired by Sir Donald Acheson, was set up in July 1997. Despite having had 18 years to have formulated policies to reduce inequalities in health, despite the abundance of evidence that the underlying causes are the increasingly unequal distributions of income and increases in poverty (which they accepted), despite the urgent need to take action to prevent excess illness and premature mortality among the poorest in Britain, the government decided it should not act until the Inquiry had reported.

However, the government constrained the Inquiry to limit the recommendations which it could make to be "within the broad framework of the Government's overall financial strategy" and to only consider the situation in England (see Box 5.1). The costing of policy suggestions and the setting of targets were also deemed to be outside the remit of the Inquiry Committee.

Box 5.1: Terms of Reference of the Independent Inquiry into Inequalities in Health

1) To moderate a Department of Health review of the latest available information on inequalities of health, using data from the Office for National Statistics, the Department of Health and elsewhere. The data review would summarise the evidence of inequalities of health and expectation of life in England and identify trends.

2) In the light of that evidence, to conduct – within the broad framework of the Government's overall financial strategy – an independent review to identify priority areas for future policy development, which scientific and expert evidence indicates are likely to offer opportunities for Government to develop beneficial, cost effective and affordable interventions to reduce health interventions.

3) The review will report to the Secretary of State for Health. The report will be published and its conclusions, based on evidence, will contribute to the development of a new strategy for health.

Source: Independent Inquiry into Inequalities in Health (1998, p 156)

The Labour government's self-imposed financial constraints were designed to maintain the confidence of the City of London and the financial markets in general in the new Labour government. However, the resulting lack of extra money reduced ministers to making press statements, led by the Secretary of State for Health, showing that they knew what the root causes of inequalities were, but not promising that they were going to address them quickly:

> Inequality in health is the worst inequality of all. There is no more serious inequality than knowing that you'll die sooner because you're badly off. (Dobson and DoH, 1997a)

The policies they claimed would help reduce health inequalities were tackling low pay, reducing unemployment and building homes, and these would be addressed through the national Minimum Wage, the 'New Deal', or Welfare to Work, and the building of new council houses. Surprisingly, they did not claim that increased spending on education would have an effect. It was not until two years after taking power that a Minimum Wage was introduced (in April 1999), at the low level of £3.60 per hour. However, the majority of those living on very low incomes are not in work and could not take work even if more jobs were available (because they are caring for children and other dependants or are over retirement age). Building homes, while necessary, does not stop people being badly off and none of these policies reduce the underlying inequalities in income, wealth and poverty that cause inequalities in health.

A month later, in September 1997, more evidence of the growth in health inequalities was released by the government (*Health inequalities*, edited by Drever and Whitehead, 1997) and, again, the government's response showed that they understood the causes of health inequalities but showed no sign of quickly tackling them:

> This report tells the tale of two Britains divided by ever widening health inequality. It shows the stark reality of a nation divided by its health i.e. the poorer and more socially deprived you are, the more likely you are to suffer ill health and die younger than those higher up the social scale. (Jowell and DoH, 1997b)

Below this soundbite, some of the first public signs of back-tracking were listed: "No one pretends that these inequalities which have been entrenched over many years can be reversed overnight. To make a real difference, we need long term policies" (Jowell and DoH, 1997b). The policies Tessa Jowell listed were the same three Frank Dobson had come up with the month before, but Welfare to Work now headed the list, followed by the Minimum Wage and then the "phased release of council receipts" to build homes. To these she added that a "strong education system will help provide the springboard to opportunity" and that "the Social Exclusion Unit will concentrate government action on bringing back into society's mainstream those whose lives are lived on the margins".

From October 1997 onwards, the government and, in particular, the Department of Health, went into a spin of policy pronouncements, for example, 'Healthy Homes for Healthy Lives, Frank Dobson addresses National Housing Federation' (Dobson and DoH, 1997b). In this speech, Dobson admitted that:

> My officials tell me it's hard to prove that better housing improves people's health. That's because it's hard to separate out the impact of housing on health from the impact of poverty, crime, and joblessness and all the other things that harm the health of most people who have nowhere decent to live. That's just another way of saying we have to tackle the lot – and that's what we are doing. Not just the

Health Department, not just Environment, Transport and the Regions.
The whole Government. (Dobson and DoH, 1997b)

In her speech at a London conference on 29 October 1997, 'Action for
health – the ultimate partnership scheme', Tessa Jowell pledged "to listen,
learn and act in partnership with health professionals, local authorities
and patients to improve public health" in preparing her Department's
Green Paper on the issue (Jowell and DoH, 1997c).

The following day, Health Minister, Alan Milburn, announced: "£30
million for new partnerships to target health inequalities" (Milburn and
DoH, 1997) and so the funding for the 'Health Action Zones' was set.
However, this £30m was for the 1999/2000 financial year. As we stated
above, during the 1998/99 financial year Health Action Zones were
only to receive an additional £4m. Thus a tiny budget was to be spent
during the first two years of Labour government on reducing inequalities
in health, but the Health Action Zones resulted in good publicity for
the government which was able to claim to be doing something.

'Partnership is the key to improving public health' was the title of
Frank Dobson's speech at the 'Healthy Plymouth' Conference on 28
November 1997 (Plymouth was later to become the only area in the
country to become a Health, Education and Employment Action Zone
all at once). In his speech, Dobson described how the partnership was
helping "people on low incomes have greater access to healthy food"
and has "checked homes for dodgy electrical wiring and promoted
smoke alarms" (Dobson and DoH, 1997c). While these may all be
thoughtful things to do, helping the poor (in selected areas only) locate
reasonable greengrocers and tidying up the wiring is unlikely to have a
major impact on reducing inequalities in health across Britain.

Health Action Zones and area-based policies

The White Paper *The new NHS – Modern and dependable*, published on 9
December 1997 (DoH, 1997) claimed that Health Action Zones would
"blaze the trail" for modernising the NHS. It said:

> Starting in up to ten areas from April 1998, they will bring together
> all those in a health authority area or wider, to improve the health of
> local people. The accent will be on partnership and innovation,
> finding new ways to tackle health problems and reshape local services.

> Health Action Zones will be concentrated in areas of pronounced
> deprivation and poor health, reflecting the Government's
> commitment to tackle entrenched inequalities. An early task for
> each Health Action Zone will be to develop clear targets, agreed
> with the NHS Executive, for measurable improvements every year.
> (DoH, 1997, 1998b)

Despite the lack of any published evidence that Health Action Zones
had met these 'clear targets', a second wave of 15 Health Action Zones
were announced on 11 August 1998 in Tees; Wakefield; Leeds; Hull and
East Riding; Merseyside (St Helens and Knowsley, Liverpool, Wirral,
Sefton); Bury and Rochdale; Nottingham; Sheffield; Leicester City;
Wolverhampton; Walsall; North Staffordshire; Cornwall; Camden and
Islington and Brent (Brent and Harrow Health Authority). Significant
additional funding of £293m for the Health Action Zones over the
three years 1999/2002 was announced on 23 April 1999 (DoH, 1999b).

John Denham (Minister for Health) has stated that "Health among
the poor must improve at a faster rate than the general population. This
means tackling ill health that results from poverty where poverty occurs"
and that "Health Action Zones are a key part of the Government's drive
in tackling health inequalities" (Denham and DoH, 1999). However,
area-based anti-inequality policies such as the action zones have a long
history of only limited successes or even outright failure. The lessons
from the 12 Community Development Projects established in 1969 in
areas of high social need appear to have been ignored (CDP, 1977).

An area-based rather than people-based approach to attacking
inequalities in health, poverty and deprivation can only ever provide
help for a relatively small minority of people since most 'poor areas'
only contain a minority of 'poor' households and a majority of 'non-
poor' households (Lee et al, 1995). For example, there are 1.1 million
people in the Tyne and Wear Health Action Zone and the majority of
them are not poor, neither do they have bad health. The criteria used
to select the areas of greatest health needs are also often very vague
(Carstairs, 1994; Taylor, 1998). Indeed, the Health Action Zones have
been allocated on the basis of competitive tender rather than purely on
the basis of greatest health needs. Thus, the government seems to have
learnt little from previous failures and has ignored "the strongly held
view of those working in regeneration and anti-poverty, that resources

should be allocated overwhelmingly according to need and not by competition" (Alcock et al, 1998).

The problem of the relative lack of effectiveness of area-based policies has been known and well documented for over 25 years (Barnes and Lucas, 1975; Townsend, 1979; Robson et al, 1994; Glennerster et al, 1999). Inequalities in health are a national problem that require national solutions. The root cause of inequalities in health is poverty which area-based policies cannot tackle effectively or efficiently. For example, in the Luton Health Action Zone, the health needs of Asian women will be particularly addressed. There will be a focus on increasing the uptake of cervical screening, the development of a community-based colposcopy service with a female consultant and a partnership between the NHS and the Asian community to address child development problems (DoH, 1998b). However, there are far more Asian women in Birmingham than in Luton and Birmingham does not have a Health Action Zone. Similarly, Plymouth Health Action Zone is developing new approaches to improving dental health, particularly in children (DoH, 1998b). Yet there are far more children with dental health needs in Bristol, Bournemouth or Brighton, which do not have Health Action Zones, than there are in Plymouth.

The Health Action Zones, like other such programmes in the past, will create a flurry of activity at relatively little cost but will probably have little lasting impact on inequalities in health (Higgens, 1998). Even if the Health Action Zones were to be successful, it is doubtful if their success could be easily replicated elsewhere since their success would inevitably be based upon local enthusiasm, energy and expertise which may not be present in many other areas (Davey Smith and Gordon, 2000: forthcoming).

Spreading the responsibility – thinly

The first new year after their election victory brought an even jollier spirit of collaboration within government:'The whole of the government tackling health inequalities – a new spirit of optimism and hope' says Frank Dobson (Dobson and DoH, 1998a). The Secretary of State explained just how much New Labour cared:

> And our commitment to reducing these massive inequalities in health isn't just a matter for the Department of Health. If it's to work, the whole of Government must play its part. And it is. The Prime

Minister is passionate about reducing these inequalities. (Dobson and DoH, 1998a)

The list of government polices that Dobson claimed were tackling inequalities in health was now in a new order: food safety and the new Foods Standards Agency came first; housing was second; traffic pollution third; Welfare to Work fourth; the minimum wage fifth; cutting VAT on fuel sixth; and he then claimed:

These are the actions the Government is taking right across the board. They will all improve the health of the people affected. They are all targeted as they should be – on the people who are worst off. So they will all help reduce inequalities in health. (Dobson and DoH, 1998a)

Just how tackling traffic pollution and improving food was to be targeted was not made clear but, in his next breath, Dobson spread the responsibility even further: "But it's not just a job for central government and the NHS. It's a job for local councils, voluntary organisations and businesses in every locality...". The responsibility and hence future blame – were inequalities not to fall following these 'targeted' policies – was all to be shared. As Dobson went on to say:

There's no need to wait for a change in the law. Local small area surveys can be done now providing useful information and showing what can be achieved. And that's really important. (Dobson and DoH, 1998a)

A week later, not to be outdone by Dobson, Jowell explained how lone parents and their children could help too: 'Minister pledges action to tackle health inequalities for lone parents and their children' (Jowell and DoH, 1998a). She acknowledged that the main cause of poor health among lone-parent families was poverty but made no mention of how her government had helped to increase their poverty through its reductions in the levels of benefits for those without work. Instead, she spelt out how they too could be encouraged to move into the world of work.

Our Healthier Nation and 'the Third Way'

All the statements above were leading up to the government's major policy announcement on public health, the 1998 Green Paper on *Our Healthier Nation: A contract for health* (DoH, 1998a) which was published two weeks later and announced to the press by Tessa Jowell on 5 February. Jowell claimed that the new health targets outlined in the Paper would underpin the government's aim of "improving the health of the worst off in society and narrowing the health gap". In fact, all of the targets could be reached even if health inequalities continued to increase, as there were no specific targets stated for the reduction of inequalities. The only actual change the Paper announced was: "a new Internet website, called Wired for Health, [which] will mean every child and teacher in the country will be able to find straight facts on health at the touch of a button" (Jowell and DoH, 1998b). Websites are relatively cheap to create and to run and their impact uncertain. They are also most easily accessible to the rich.

Many of the remarks by government officials on health and health inequalities highlighted the need for 'listening', 'learning', and 'partnership'. However, the voices of those suffering most from inequality were little heard. Finally, in the press release that announced the Green Paper, the Department of Health gave the response from the public. To advertise the Green Paper they paraded Derrick Evans, better known as 'Mr Motivator', the leotard-clad fitness instructor of the ITV Breakfast show GMTV. However, the use of Mr Motivator was perhaps relevant as government policies were beginning to move back towards ideas of individual responsibility:

> To achieve these aims [including narrowing the health gap], the Government is setting out a third way between the old extremes of individual victim blaming on the one hand and nanny state social engineering on the other. Good health is no longer about blame, but about opportunity and responsibility. Our third way is a national contract for better health. Under this contract, the Government, local communities and individuals will join in partnership to improve all our health. (Jowell and DoH, 1998b)

So, by the first anniversary of their landslide election victory, New Labour, through its ministers, had moved away from the collective responsibility they first espoused upon gaining office as well as from their understanding of the causes of health inequalities, pronounced publicly less than a year before. The causes were no longer primarily poverty – the individual actions of the disadvantaged were just as important under the new (third) way.

The Independent Inquiry into Inequalities in Health

The report of the Independent Inquiry into Inequalities in Health was finally published at the end of November 1998. This was to be a landmark occasion in the field of health inequalities research and policy, arguably the most important event since the publication of the Black Report almost 20 years earlier (DHSS, 1980). However, while the new report was welcomed and contained a comprehensive review of current knowledge on the extent and trends in health inequalities, it was not the definitive document that would set the government into action as many had hoped. Surprisingly little media coverage and debate ensued but three key criticisms were levied at the report (Davey Smith et al, 1998a).

The first criticism was that there was not adequate prioritisation among the 39 sets of recommendations. Thus, the fundamental role of poverty and income differentials was lost in a sea of (albeit worthy) recommendations ranging from traffic curbing to the fluoridation of the water supply. Sir Donald Acheson, Chair of the Inquiry, responded to this remark by stating that the following three areas were considered by the scientific advisory group as crucial:

- all policies likely to have an impact on health should be evaluated in terms of their impact on health inequalities;
- a high priority should be given to the health of families with children;
- further steps should be taken to reduce income inequalities and improve the living standards of poor households (Acheson, 1998).

In the Inquiry's report there was no statement as to how the first priority listed above was to be achieved. Nor were the steps that had apparently already taken place to improve the living standards of the poor listed.

The second, and related, criticism of the Inquiry's report was that many of the recommendations were simply too vague and decontextualised to be useful. For example, the advocacy of public transport without reference to the price-increasing effects of recent privatisation policies was of little practical use.

The third set of criticisms of the report related more directly to the implementation of the recommendations: the costing of the suggested policies. As the recommendations of the report (unlike the Black Report) were not costed, it was impossible to weigh up the costs, benefits and opportunity costs of implementation or inaction. It was thus also impossible to judge the extent to which these suggestions are 'cost-effective', as the remit for the Inquiry requested. (The 1982 and 1996 costs of meeting the principal recommendations of the Black Report on inequalities of health have since been estimated by Black et al [1999] and these are included in the Preface of this book.)

The government's immediate response to the report was another press release. This time, Frank Dobson stated that: "the whole Government, led from the top by the Prime Minister, is committed to the greatest ever reduction in health inequalities" (Dobson and DoH, 1998b). He went on to concentrate on the tax and benefit changes Labour had made. However, the Minimum Wage only applied to people in work and the benefit improvements were only for families with children. He then reeled off the same list of other government policies as before.

Saving lives – the government response

Finally, in July 1999, eight months after the publication of the *Independent Inquiry into Inequalities in Health*, the government responded with a White Paper on public health (*Saving lives: Our healthier nation*, DoH 1999a) and an Action Report on *Reducing health inequalities* (DoH, 1999c). Somewhat surprisingly, and reminiscent of the Black Report's publication of 20 years previously, the White Paper was made widely available via The Stationery Office shops around the country but the Action Report was only available from the Department of Health, which guaranteed it a much more restricted circulation.

The Action Report represents a response to the recommendations made by the Independent Inquiry into Inequalities in Health. It details plans to cut the number of people sleeping rough by two thirds by 2002 and to halve the rate of conception among under 18s in England by 2010. It told of how officials are discussing with the food industry the possibility of reducing salt levels in processed food and the Social Exclusion Unit is examining ways of improving shopping access in deprived areas. A week's course of nicotine replacement therapy is to be provided free to all the poorest smokers. Government-funded researchers are investigating why fewer poor mothers breast feed and infant feeding advisers have been appointed to increase the prevalence of breast feeding. Resource packs will be provided to schools to increase awareness of healthy eating under the healthy schools initiative, school breakfast clubs are to be encouraged and research is to be conducted to establish practical ways of encouraging children to eat fruit and vegetables. National nutritional standards for school meals will be re-established at some point in the future (DoH, 1999a; Burke, 1999).

However, while these are all laudable plans, they are very unlikely to have a major impact on health inequalities at a national level.

The White Paper set clear and unambiguous targets for improving "the health of the population as a whole". Targets to be achieved by the year 2010 include reducing the death rate in people aged under 75 years from coronary heart disease by at least two fifths; from cancers by a fifth; from accidents by a tenth; and from mental illness by a fifth. The total number of deaths from these causes is to be reduced by 300,000 over the next 10 years. A budget of £96m has been allocated to these programmes through a public health development fund over the next three years.

However, none of this £96m has been allocated to reducing health inequalities, nor did the White Paper set any national targets for reducing health inequalities. Instead of national targets with clear and unambiguous goals on inequalities in health, the White Paper requires health authorities to set their own local targets. These local targets for reducing the health divide are to be met from the health authorities' existing funds. Despite the fact that the White Paper claims that its goals are "consistent with the World Health Organisation (Europe)'s new programme for the 21st Century *Health 21*", to which the United Kingdom is a signatory, the government was clearly unwilling to include Target 2 of the *Health 21* strategy in the White Paper. Target 2 states: "By the year 2020, the health gap between socio-economic groups within countries should be reduced by at least one quarter in all member states, by substantially improving the level of health of disadvantaged groups" (WHO Europe, 1999). This is not even a particularly ambitious target on reducing health inequalities but it is clearly more ambitious than the British government is currently prepared to commit itself to.

The problem of poverty and the problem of riches

We are not arguing that New Labour have done nothing, nor that they do not want to end inequalities in health. Instead, we believe that what they have done will be relatively ineffective and that if they are serious about achieving their goal of reducing inequalities in health more fundamental policies – of the kind they have advocated in the past and when in opposition – need to be implemented. Almost all the senior cabinet members, including the Prime Minister, have repeatedly spoken about the overriding need to end poverty. Gordon Brown and Robin Cook, who edited and wrote chapters in a book on poverty in Scotland (1983), have stated again and again how they want to end poverty both in Britain and in other countries. They are not lying or trying to be deliberately misleading – they really do mean what they say. The problem is not mendaciousness but 'practical politics'. Labour politicians do not believe they can be sure of re-election if they raise taxes for the rich and perhaps they think that there are very few votes in reducing unfairness in people's health chances.

'New Labour' differs from 'Old Labour' in that it has abandoned the rhetoric of 'democratic socialism' and now acts as a purely 'social democratic' party. Translated, this means that New Labour has completely abandoned the concept of the 'problem of riches'. As we briefly discussed in Chapter 1, Gordon Brown's conclusions to his and Robin Cook's overview of *Scotland: The real divide* in 1983 showed this concept was one they previously understood well, as:

> This would mean restoring to the centre of the tax system two basic principles: the first, that those who cannot afford to pay tax should not have to pay it; and the second, that taxation should rise progressively with income. Programmes that merely redistribute poverty from families to single persons, from the old to the young, from the sick to the healthy, are not a solution. What is needed, is a programme of reform that ends the current situation where the top 10% own 80% of our wealth and 30% of income, even after tax. As Tawney remarked, 'What some people call the problem of poverty, others call the problem of riches'. (Brown and Cook, 1983, p 22)

However, Gordon Brown, in his modern guise, believes in the New Labour policy of trying to create more millionaires. Old Labour could end poverty very quickly (at least in theory) by raising the extra money needed for the poor by redistribution: as Denis Healey said, "by taxing the rich till the pips squeak". New Labour believes that taking money from the rich and/or middle classes is political suicide (at least if it is done too obviously through raising direct taxes). They believe that John Major won the election in 1992 because of John Smith's pledge to raise income taxes and concluded that the rich must be allowed to keep their money.

Therefore, New Labour can only raise the money necessary to end poverty from redistributing any extra money arising from economic growth and this is a relatively slow process. This has been so particularly when Gordon Brown committed Labour to keeping to the Conservative's spending plans for the first two years of office. This is the reason why the anti-poverty policies which they have announced are relatively ineffective as they are all attempts to alleviate poverty which do not cost much money. For example, the Social Exclusion Unit's remit covers 18 worthy causes (including rough sleeping, truancy, school exclusions, teenage pregnancy, community self-help, neighbourhood wardens and unpopular housing) but the Unit has no budget and does not consider income inequality. Poverty really is a problem of the lack of enough money – if you give poor people enough money they stop being poor – it is as simple as that.

New Labour believes that the voting public is simply not prepared to pay the price for ending poverty and inequalities in health if it means that taxes have to be raised.

Politics, public opinion and poverty reduction

To generate sufficient political momentum for additional anti-poverty expenditure, informed opinion must be unanimous on the necessity of reducing inequality and poverty in order to effectively tackle problems of inequalities in health. Both the Black and Acheson Committees into Inequalities in Health stressed the overriding need to reduce childhood poverty. After 20 years of research on social and economic change and increasing average incomes and wealth in Britain, the key recommendations by expert committees on how to reduce inequalities in health remain essentially the same.

Widespread public support is also a necessary requirement for achieving extra anti-poverty expenditure and the public's support for such policies is evident. The rapid growth of inequality and poverty in Britain during the 1980s resulted in major shifts in public opinion. By 1986, the British Social Attitudes Survey found that 87% of people thought that the government 'definitely should' or 'probably should' spend more money to get rid of poverty'. In 1989, the European Union-wide Eurobarometer opinion survey found that British people thought the 'fight against poverty' ranked second only to 'world peace' in the list of great causes worth taking risks and making sacrifices for (Eurobarometer, 1989). This view was widely held across the then 12 member countries of the European Union (Table 5.1).

Table 5.1: Worthwhile great causes in the UK and Europe (1989)

Question: *'In your opinion, in this list which are the great causes which nowadays are worth the trouble of taking risks and making sacrifices for?'*

(Answers in order of preference)	UK (%)	The 12 EC countries (%)
World peace	71	75
The fight against poverty	57	57
Human rights	55	60
Protection of wildlife	48	57
Freedom of the individual	43	39
Defence of the country	41	30
The fight against racism	32	36
Sexual equality	25	25
My religious faith	18	19
The unification of Europe	9	18
The revolution	2	5
None of these	2	1
No reply	1	2

Source: Eurobarometer (1989)

The two *Breadline Britain* surveys recorded the change in the public's attitude to the government's response to the problem of poverty (Gordon and Pantazis, 1997). In both the 1983 and 1990 studies, the following question was asked: 'Still thinking about people who lack the things you have said are necessities for living in Britain today, do you think that the government is doing too much, too little or about the right amount to help these people?'. The results are presented in Table 5.2.

Table 5.2: Is the government doing enough for the poor?

	1983 (%) n=1,174	1990 (%) n=1,831
Too much	6	5
Too little	57	70
About the right amount	33	18
Don't know	4	7

Source: Analysis by authors of the *Breadline Britain* surveys (1983 and 1990)

Table 5.2 shows how public opinion changed between 1983 and 1990. There was a remarkable shift in public opinion among those considering that the government was doing 'too little' to help. In 1983, 57% thought too little was being done but, by 1990, 70% of respondents thought this. There was a concomitant decline in the percentage of respondents who thought the government was doing 'about the right amount', with the numbers thinking that the government was doing 'too much' remaining relatively constant. This shift in public attitudes resulted from the greater visibility of the problems of deprivation as the numbers living in poverty increased during the 1980s.

Given the evidence shown in Table 5.2, it is unsurprising that there is no evidence of any increase in the numbers of people who are strongly opposed to reducing the income differences between the rich and the poor. The British Social Attitudes Survey has asked a representative sample of the British population about this issue in 1985, 1986, 1990 and 1996 as part of an International Social Science Programme questionnaire on the role of governments. The percentage of the British population who believed that the government 'definitely should not' act to reduce income inequality was 10% in 1985, 8.2% in 1986, 9.4% in 1990 and 9.8% in 1996. However, it must be noted that, although only 10% of the British population oppose policies to reduce inequality, this 10% is likely to contain some very vocal and powerful (and very probably wealthy) people. Throughout the 1980s and in the 1990s, the views of this 10% of the population prevailed and the wishes of the majority were ignored.

Criticism of government inaction on poverty carries little weight unless people are prepared to pay for the costs of change. Both the 1983 and 1990 *Breadline Britain* surveys asked respondents two questions to see how much they were willing to pay to help those living in need:

Q9a: 'If the government proposed to increase income tax by one penny (1p) in the pound to enable everyone to afford the items you have said are necessities, on balance would you support or oppose this policy?'

and

Q9b: 'If the government proposed to increase income tax by five pence (5p) in the pound to enable everyone to afford the items you have said are necessities, on balance would you support or oppose this policy?'

Table 5.3: **Change in public opinion about income tax increases to help alleviate poverty between 1983 and 1990 in Britain**

	Opinion on a 1p in the £ income tax increase		Opinion on a 5p in the £ income tax increase	
	1983	1990	1983	1990
Support	74	75	34	43
Oppose	20	18	53	44
Don't know	6	7	13	13

Source: Analysis by authors of the *Breadline Britain* surveys (1983 and 1990)

In both 1983 and 1990, approximately three quarters of respondents (74% in 1983 and 75% in 1990) supported a 1p in the pound income tax increase. There was a significant shift in public attitudes among those supporting a 5p in the pound income tax increase. In 1990, almost as many respondents supported a 5p rise (43%) as opposed it (44%), whereas, in 1983, only 34% had supported such a large income tax increase.

By 1990, there was a remarkable level of agreement across all divisions in society that the government should increase income tax by 1p in the pound to help alleviate poverty. Even 70% of Conservative supporters agreed with this policy when interviewed. However, in the Budget of March 1999, the Labour government pledged to cut the basic rate of income tax by 1p in the pound.

Recently, Milton Keynes Unitary Council conducted a referendum on how large an increase there ought to be in the Council Tax. Between 1 and 19 February 1999, 66,647 people voted (a turnout of 44.7%) on three budget options:

- Option 1, a 15% Council Tax increase (six times the rate of inflation)
- Option 2, a 9.8% Council Tax increase (four times the rate of inflation)
- Option 3, a 5% Council Tax increase (twice the rate of inflation).

Only 30% voted for the lowest 5% increase in Council Tax, with 70% voting for either the 9.8% or 15% increase (Milton Keynes Council, 1999). The voters of Milton Keynes, when given the option, voted for substantial increases in their taxes in order to provide for better local authority services. The turnout of 44.7% for the Budget Referendum was larger than the turnout for any of the annual Milton Keynes local council elections held during the previous five years.

Given the British public's support for poverty alleviation policies and their apparent willingness to pay extra taxes to fund these policies, it is not surprising that many senior Labour politicians, including the Prime Minister, highlighted the need to tackle the problems of poverty in the run up to the 1997 General Election. Indeed, the government Green Paper on Welfare Reform (*New ambitions for our country: A new contract for welfare*) published in March 1998 (DSS, 1998b), emphasised the need to tackle "the scourge of child poverty" and "support all families with children, especially poorer families" (DSS, 1998b). The solution to poverty proposed in the Green Paper is through 'work for those who can' and 'security for those cannot'. Neither voters, government ministers nor those concerned with public health want to see a continuation of the growth in inequality and poverty that occurred in the 1980s and 1990s.

The only way that inequalities in health can be tackled is to also tackle the wider problems of inequality in society. There is no new medicine, treatment or 'technical' fix that would allow the widening health gap to be narrowed while poverty remains at its current high level. There is huge public support to reduce poverty and to pay through higher taxes to achieve this.

Redistribution by stealth?

New Labour's nervousness about alienating 'middle England' by increasing direct taxes has led many commentators to believe that Gordon Brown has attempted to redistribute income by stealth, using indirect taxation and other budgetary measures to take money from the 'rich' and give it to the 'poor'. The 1999 Labour Budget was hailed by many as a brilliant *tour de force* by the Chancellor that redistributed income in a relatively painless manner and would help alleviate the scourge of child poverty. It was the first Labour Budget that was not constrained by the self-imposed requirement to maintain the spending limits laid down by the previous Conservative administration. A number of dramatic measures were introduced designed to help families with children; these included:

- the introduction of the 10p income tax band;
- the abolition of the Married Couple's Allowance (MCA) and the Additional Personal Allowance (APA);
- the introduction of the Children's Tax Credit.

Both the Microsimulation Unit in the Department of Applied Economics at the University of Cambridge and the Institute of Fiscal Studies have modelled the redistributional effects of these changes and have come to similar conclusions. Table 5.4 shows the combined impact of these Budget measures on the distribution of family incomes. The proportions of families gaining or losing are shown for each decile, which divide the population into 10 equal-sized income groups (Sutherland, 1999).

Table 5.4: **Percentage of gainers and losers by income decile: three Finance Bill changes**

Income decile group	All families	
	Gainers	**Losers**
Poorest	1	1
2	7	3
3	21	4
4	39	6
5	63	10
6	73	13
7	73	19
8	71	25
9	66	32
Richest	57	41
All	47	16

Source: Sutherland (1999)

The results in Table 5.4 are clear – overall, 47% of families gained on average about £1 per week from the budgetary changes and 16% of families were made worse off. However, among the poorest 10% of families in the bottom decile of the income distribution, 1% of families gained and 1% were made worse off, leaving 98% of the poorest families unaffected by these budgetary changes. On average, most people gained from the Budget, particularly families with children. However, among the families with the lowest incomes, a few families with children gained at the expense of poor families without children.

During the 1980s, as we outlined above, Gordon Brown and Robin Cook (1983) argued that: "Programmes that merely redistribute poverty from families to single persons, from the old to the young, from the sick to the healthy, are not a solution." (p 22). Unfortunately, this was precisely the effect of the main 1999 Finance Bill changes.

There have now been three Labour Budgets since their landslide election victory in May 1997 which have introduced a large number of taxation, government spending and welfare benefit changes. The key word used by Chancellor Gordon Brown in relation to all these three budgets has been 'fairness'. Figure 5.1 shows the percentage of gainers and losers following all the changes made in the past three Labour Budgets (Immervoll et al, 1999).

Figure 5.1: **Percentage of gainers and losers following three Labour Budgets**

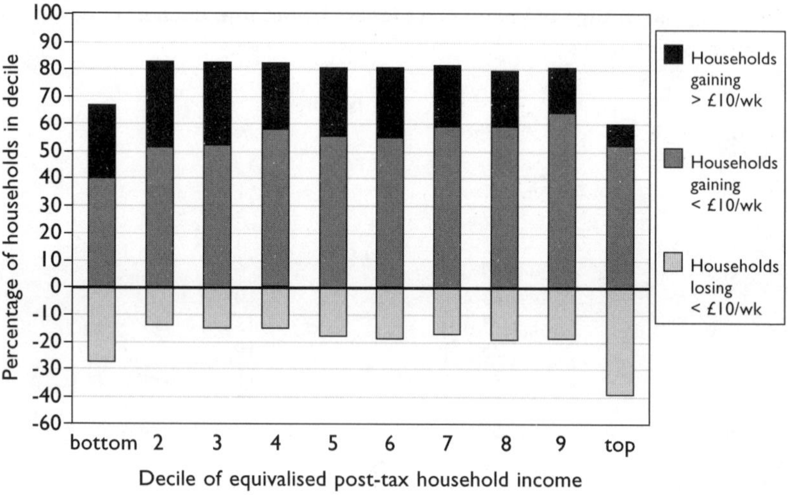

Source: Immervoll et al (1999)

Again, the results are clear – the overwhelming majority of households are better off as a result of the changes made in the past three Labour Budgets. On average, households in every income decile have shared in the growing wealth of the country. However, there have been losers as well as gainers, as Figure 5.1 shows. Overall, 80% of households are better off and 20% are worse off, but the largest proportion of losers are among the poorest (28.1%) and the richest (39.2%). More than a quarter of households in the lowest income group are poorer as the result of three Labour Budgets. It is questionable if this would be considered to be a 'fair' result by the average voter. Income has been redistributed by Labour but not all the poor have gained, indeed, many middle-income households have done better out of the budget changes than have poor households, particularly poor households dependent on welfare benefits.

To put this somewhat depressing picture into perspective, the Labour Budgets have been vastly more progressive than the previous Conservative Budgets. The last Conservative Budget, in 1996, redistributed money from the poor to the rich as previous Conservative Budgets had done (Chadwick et al, 1997). The past three Labour Budgets have introduced a number of welcome and progressive changes but, in total, they have done relatively little to reduce the huge inequalities in wealth and health that exist in Britain today.

Reducing inequalities in health

It is clear that the most effective way of reducing inequalities in health in Britain is to reduce poverty. The poor have too little money and the solution to ending their poverty is to provide them with more money. As we repeatedly argue, poverty reduction really is something that can be achieved by 'throwing money at the problem'. However, this solution requires a degree of political will and support that may not be currently achievable and some ways of spending money are obviously more effective than others.

The government's preferred method of alleviating poverty is through providing training and coercion to get unemployed people into jobs. In September 1993, a Ditchley Park seminar on Inequalities in Health organised by the King's Fund, concluded that "no strategy to tackle health inequalities will be worthy of the name if it is not committed to reducing unemployment to the lowest possible level" (Benzeval et al, 1995). However, the current government employment strategy has two major flaws. Firstly, no amount of help, advice and training can reduce unemployment if there are no jobs available. Policies are needed that are designed to increase the supply of jobs. Secondly, there are large numbers of poor households for which employment does not represent a way out of poverty, for example, the retired, people with full-time caring responsibilities and the permanently sick.

Poverty can be reduced by raising the standard of living of poor people through the provision of better central and local government and voluntary services or by providing income 'in kind' rather than 'in cash'. A comprehensive anti-poverty policy needs to encompass both ways of increasing the cash incomes of poor people as well as simultaneously raising their standard of living via the provision of better 'in kind' services.

Social policy researchers and economists have proposed a range of affordable and cost-effective anti-poverty policies. Policies aimed at increasing the standard of living and incomes of poor families with children, of disabled people and of elderly people will have the greatest impact on rapidly reducing inequalities in health. The quickest and most cost-effective method of alleviating poverty is to increase the value of welfare benefits and pensions and improve public services and social housing. A number of specific policies will be discussed in the next section.

Economists have also designed and costed a number of 'affordable' Basic Income schemes that, if properly implemented, would effectively end poverty in Britain (Desai, 1998). A Basic Income is a payment received by every person or household that provides a minimum income and the amount is based only on age and family status but is otherwise unconditional.

There are three main advantages claimed for Basic Income schemes (Brittan and Webb, 1990):

- They should plug the gaps and loopholes in social security and reduce the number of people living in poverty.
- They should remove the unemployment and poverty traps that result from the high rates of benefit withdrawal when the unemployed obtain work, or people with low incomes move up the earnings ladder.
- They are desirable because people should have a means of subsistence independent of needs and not dependent on complicated contribution records or intrusive scrutiny of personal means.

Most existing social security benefits in industrialised countries are contingent, which means that they are related to misfortune or conditions such as age, sickness or unemployment. By contrast, a Basic Income depends only on very general characteristics, such as number of dependants. There are no questions or conditions relating to effort to find work, state of health, contribution records or capital holdings. Basic Incomes could replace many existing specific social security benefits. There would always be people with special needs requiring extra sums on a conditional or discretionary basis but fewer cases than at present. Some advocates believe that Basic Income payments should take the form of a tax credit to be set off against tax but received as a positive payment from the state by those with insufficient tax liabilities. The current government is implementing some of these policies – if only in a very limited way.

As an example, the government has implemented legislation to provide a guaranteed minimum income for working families with children of £180 per week from April 1999, increasing to £190 per week in October 1999. Pensioners have also had a guaranteed minimum income of £75 for single people and £117 for couples since April 1999. Similarly, severely disabled people who are unable to work have been guaranteed a minimum income of £128 per week. However, these proposals do not go much beyond existing levels of Income Support and Family Credit and, like all existing means-tested benefits, will fail to reach large numbers of those legally entitled to those benefits. In practice, the proposals will make little difference to existing living standards especially when, as in the case of Incapacity Benefit, the government is proposing to save more money in cuts, than they are prepared to spend on the additions to selected means-tested benefits for severely disabled adults and young children.

The political will clearly does not presently exist to implement a broad-based minimum income guarantee for the whole population at a sufficient level to end poverty. For a government supposedly committed to new thinking, claiming to be innovative and to have broken from the shackles of the past, the fact that it is not willing to countenance a novel approach such as Basic Income schemes is a serious disappointment. In the absence of a comprehensive approach, as a second-best by some distance, a number of specific targeted policies could be implemented that would reduce poverty among elderly, sick and disabled people and families with children. These would also have the effect of leading to some reduction in inequalities in health.

The importance of services

Most 'economic' studies of poverty ignore the importance of services in raising the standard of living of poor households. This failure often makes international comparisons of poverty rates based on cash incomes alone of only limited value. The services (in-kind benefits) provided by the welfare state, such as the NHS, state education and local government services, have a greater effect on increasing the standard of living of the lowest income households than do the combined values of their wages and salaries, Income Support and the retirement pensions available to those households. Table 5.5 shows the contribution that earnings, cash benefits and in-kind services had on the poorest and richest 10% of all UK households in 1996-97.

Table 5.5: Income, taxes and benefit contribution to the average incomes of the poorest and richest 10% of households in the UK in 1996-97

Income	Poorest 10% of households (*n*=2,425,000)	Richest 10% of households (*n*=2,425,000)
Wages and salaries	1,026	36,599
Other income	822	18,762
Total income	**1,848**	**55,361**
Retirement pension	1,227	506
Income Support	1,205	6
Child Benefit	434	141
Housing Benefit	536	8
Other cash benefits	766	245
Total cash benefits	**4,168**	**906**
Direct taxes (income, council, etc)	719	13,166
Total disposable income	**5,297**	**43,101**
Indirect taxes (VAT, etc)	1,926	5,916
Post tax income	3,371	37,184
Benefits in kind		
NHS	1,894	1,240
Education	1,959	385
Other benefits in kind	210	165
Total benefits in kind	**4,063**	**1,790**
Final income	7,433	38,974

Source: Analysis by authors of data in *Economic trends* and *Social trends*

Table 5.5 shows that the richest 10% of households in the UK have an average final income of £38,974 (after accounting for the contribution of benefits and the effects of taxation), which is more than five times larger than the average final income of the poorest 10% of households (eg £7,433). It also illustrates the huge importance of services to the poorest households. Over half of the income (£4,063) that the poorest 10% of households receive is in the form of 'benefits in kind'. The poorest households each received on average £1,894 worth of services from the NHS alone, which represents over a quarter of their final income. If the NHS was not a free service, the poorest households would be 25% poorer. The contribution of NHS services to the final income of the poorest 10% of retired households (629,000 households) is even greater. They received £2,639 worth of NHS services each on average in 1996-97, which represented almost half of their final incomes of £5,475 per year.

Table 5.5 illustrates the effectiveness of the welfare state system in alleviating poverty. Cash and in-kind benefits raise the real incomes of the poorest households from £1,848 to a final income of £7,433, a fourfold increase. This was not a sufficient amount to raise the poorest 10% of households out of poverty, which would have required approximately a five to sixfold increase in original income in 1996-97. However, the welfare state prevented the poorest households from sinking into a state of absolute destitution. There is no doubt that, properly funded, the welfare state system in Britain could be used to rapidly bring an end to poverty and begin to reduce inequalities in health.

Equity in service delivery

Given the importance of in-kind services in alleviating poverty, there has been surprisingly little work done on equity in service delivery. Many researchers have assumed that, since many welfare state services are free at the point of use (like the NHS and most education services) or are eligibility or means-tested, they must be going to the people with greatest needs.

As Table 5.5 demonstrates, the NHS and local government represent a substantial part of the overall welfare state in Britain and are particularly important in the provision of services in-kind as opposed to cash benefits. Until the 1980s, our knowledge of the distribution of such benefits in kind had been very patchy but recent surveys, including many carried out by MORI for individual local authorities, have provided a fuller picture. The central question motivating these studies has been whether local public services are an effective mechanism of redistribution in favour of the 'poor' and disadvantaged or whether many of these services are in fact used more by the better off.

The *Breadline Britain* surveys examined both the use of a range of services by different socio-economic groups and also asked respondents to indicate which of these services they believed to be essential rather than just desirable (Table 5.6).

Table 5.6 shows that a majority of a representative sample of the British public regard all these services as essential. For all bar two of these services, the proportion is around 80% or more. Only museums and galleries are not regarded by a substantial majority as essential and even here there is a small majority supporting this proposition. Even in the more leisure-oriented services of libraries and sports, the majorities for treating these as essential are very large. For bus services, children's services and those for elderly and disabled people, the support is overwhelming (Bramley, 1997).

Table 5.6: **Proportion of respondents regarding selected local services as essential and desirable in the 1990 *Breadline Britain* survey (%)**

Service	Essential	Desirable
Libraries	79	20
Sports and swimming	79	20
Museums and galleries	52	47
Adult evening classes	70	28
Bus services	96	2
Childcare	90	9
Play facilities	92	7
School meals	87	11
Home help	95	2
Meals on wheels	93	4
Special transport	95	2

Source: Analysis by authors of the *Breadline Britain* survey, 1990

Table 5.7 shows the usage rates and usage ratios of the 11 local public services shown in Table 5.6 by social class and poverty group ('non-poor' versus 'poor'). The first five services shown in Table 5.6 are open to all and are essentially demand-led (Bramley and Le Grand, 1992). Apart from bus services, use of these services shows a pro-rich bias to varying degrees. This characteristic is rather typical of demand-led services. They represent normal economic goods, mainly in the leisure field, of which 'better off' people generally want to and are able to consume more. Although they are free or subsidised, there are some costs involved in using them, including entry charges in some cases and the time and money costs of gaining access to them.

Table 5.7: **Usage rates and standardised usage ratios by class and deprivation for 11 local services**

Service	Usage rate (%)	Usage ratio by class	Usage ratio by poverty group
Libraries	64	1.40	1.36
Sports and swimming	55	1.34	1.19
Museums and galleries	39	2.03	1.56
Adult evening classes	22	1.88	1.52
Bus services	67	0.77	0.85
Childcare	61	0.92	1.26
Play facilities	62	0.93	1.31
School meals	52	0.70	0.79
Home help	10	0.62	0.84
Meals on wheels	5	0.32	0.57
Special transport	10	0.29	0.94

Note: Usage ratios are the ratio between the usage rate for the most advantaged group and that for the least advantaged group, with four class groups, and two poverty groups.
Source: Analysis by authors from the *Breadline Britain* survey, 1990

It is clear that the 'poor' make significantly less use of local public services in the leisure field, the difference being of the order of 20% to 50%. These services are not only failing to compensate for other deprivations but problems of access to them are, on balance, worsening the deprivation of some households. Another way of looking at these services, in particular, is that they represent examples of 'participating in the normal life of the community'. The evidence suggests that 'multiply deprived' households are less likely to participate in this 'normal life of the community'. The patterns of use in Table 5.7 are broadly consistent with those found in local authority surveys.

Bus services, school meals, home helps, meals on wheels and special transport services all demonstrate a pro-poor bias. However, this bias in favour of poorer households is not always very large. Poor households are only 5% to 20% more likely than other households to use buses, home helps or special transport. This is despite the fact that because they are less likely to own cars, or to afford private domestic service, their need is clearly considerably greater than that of richer families.

In the 1980s, research in Cheshire highlighted social care services for elderly and disabled people as the main examples of strongly 'pro-poor' services (Bramley et al, 1989). The more recent comparative work, using MORI local surveys, modified this conclusion slightly by suggesting that the pro-poor character of these services could not be taken completely for granted. It depended in part on the rationing criteria used, given that these are broadly in the category of 'needs rationed services' (Bramley, 1990; Bramley and Smart, 1993).

As mentioned, the fact that home help and special transport services are only slightly more likely to be used by poorer households is a rather surprising finding given the much greater need of poor retired people for these services. This implies that targeting is ineffective or that the criteria used to allocate these services are inadequate. We are not suggesting that targeting should be 'tightened' – rather, that it is, by its nature, inefficient.

There is also evidence that, in some areas of healthcare, disproportionately more health resources go to 'richer' households than to 'poorer' households, given the health inequalities that exist and define their relative needs. There is a range of evidence suggesting that better off, middle-class people receive more primary care and acute health services relative to need than do the poor (Chaturvedi and Ben-Shlomo, 1995, 1997; Ben-Shlomo and Chaturvedi, 1995; Worral et al, 1997; Majeed et al, 1994). However, virtually no health authorities or hospital trusts have analysed records of who is receiving their services by this method, or looked to see whether those in the greatest need are receiving the most health services. Surprisingly, much of the research into inequalities in access to healthcare does not take account of, or adjust for, need or socio-economic factors (Goddard and Smith, 1998). One of the key policies the NHS could adopt which would help reduce inequalities in health would be to perform regular equity audits and then redirect services to the 'poorest' communities that are not currently receiving adequate healthcare. It is time that the Inverse Care Law – "the availability of good medical care tends to vary inversely with the need for it in the population served" – first identified by Dr Julian Tudor Hart in 1971, was consigned to history (Tudor Hart, 1971).

Equity was one of the founding principles of the NHS and the report of the Independent Inquiry into Inequalities in Health has recommended that providing equitable access to effective care in relation to need should be a governing principle of all policies in the NHS. However, the equity should be on the basis of needs – those who are most ill should be getting most service. Priority should be given to the achievement of equity in the planning, implementation and delivery of services at every level of the NHS. The report also recommended that Directors of Public Health, working on behalf of health and local authorities, produce an equity profile for the population they serve, and undertake a triennial audit of progress towards achieving objectives to reduce inequalities in health. These policies and principles need to be adopted for both health service and local authority service provision.

However, even if good practice on equitable service delivery was adopted by the NHS and local authorities, these changes alone would not be sufficient to end inequalities in health. Other policies designed to raise the incomes of poor families with children, sick and disabled people and elderly people will also be needed and some of these are outlined in the sections that follow.

Child poverty and health

The experience of poverty and deprivation during childhood can have lifelong consequences on health. One of the most worrying aspects of the growth in poverty and inequality over the past 20 years has been the very high rates of poverty experienced by lone-parent families, families with young children, and large families (Adelman and Bradshaw, 1998). To reduce inequalities in health for children now, and for when they reach adulthood in the future, the following policies should be adopted now:

- To reduce inequalities in child health it is essential that all pregnant women are able to afford an adequate diet. Budget Standards research at the University of York (Bradshaw, 1993; Oldfield and Yu, 1993) and Loughborough (Middleton et al, 1996) indicates that the current maternity allowance is insufficient to achieve this aim. The abolition of the universal maternity allowance was a retrograde step. Maternity entitlements need to be increased, particularly for women dependent on Income Support and/or in low paid jobs.
- A third of all children live in families dependent on Income Support (Hills, 1998). The Income Support scale rates are therefore one of the most crucial factors that determine the amount of child poverty in Britain. These are currently so low that families with children will eventually sink into poverty if they become dependent on Income Support for any length of time. Additional benefits are required to support families with children.
- Approximately a quarter of all children are born to mothers under 25 years old. Therefore, the supposition that people aged less than 25 require lower rates of benefit than those over 25 needs to be re-examined urgently.
- Adequate additional benefits are needed by lone parents following the abolition of the Lone Parent premium. Lone-parent families face additional financial and time costs compared with two-parent

households and the level of benefits available to lone-parent families needs to adequately reflect these additional costs.

• Means-tested benefits are a socially divisive, costly and inefficient method of alleviating poverty as they rarely can achieve better than 80% take-up rates (Oorschot, 1995; Cordon, 1995). Universal Child Benefit rates should therefore be increased by far more than the increases announced in the 1999 Budget.

Although increasing the value of benefits available to families with children is the most important social policy for reducing poverty and inequalities in health, there are also a number of specific policies of secondary importance which will also help reduce child poverty and childhood deaths and illness.

• The rent limit on Housing Benefit needs to be removed for families with children and increased building of social housing is required to end the need for 'Bed & Breakfast' accommodation. Subsidies for Social Housing would also enable real rent levels to be reduced and the reliance on the private sector to be removed.

• The mortality rate of pedestrians in road traffic accidents (RTAs) in Britain is one of the highest in the industrialised world. Pedestrian child deaths and injury due to RTAs have a steep poverty gradient. An immediate and rigid enforcement of the speed limits in residential areas would be the most rapid and inexpensive means of reducing inequalities in health. The law needs to be enforced and the technology to achieve this (traffic calming measures, speed cameras, etc) is both readily available and relatively cheap. Speed traps might well prove to be income-generating.

• Nutritional standards for school meals have now been reintroduced but new technology (eg smart cards) needs to be employed to remove the stigma from free school meals. Free school meals entitlement should be extended to families receiving Family Credit (now Working Families Tax Credit) and free school milk provision should be made mandatory. School breakfast schemes should be examined and, where successful, be extended.

• The imprisonment and criminalisation of parents for non-payment of debt, particularly TV licence offences (Pantazis and Gordon, 1997), should cease.

• Social work and health worker practice needs to become much more poverty sensitive. Recent reviews of research on good practice for improving the health of poor families concluded with three key recommendations. Firstly, any health and welfare strategy that aims to improve family health and the ability of families to meet their own needs should have family poverty as its central concern. Local and health authorities need to ensure that staff who are likely to come into contact with poor people are trained to ensure that they are receiving their full entitlement to welfare benefits (Betts, 1993). Secondly, interagency collaboration should be a fundamental aspect of any strategy that aims to tackle the health and welfare concerns of the poor. Thirdly, parents want the opportunity to care for family health in partnership with health and welfare workers (Blackburn, 1991).

Elderly people and pensions

Elderly people are clearly more likely to die or be ill than any other group. Poverty in old age exacerbates this situation. Poor pensioners are more likely to become sick or disabled than richer pensioners and, if they become ill, poor pensioners are more likely to die younger (Arber and Ginn, 1993). The most effective way of alleviating poverty among elderly people is through pensions policy. Barbara Castle and others have recently proposed that:

> The Government should fulfil its Manifesto commitment to make the basic state pensions, the foundation of its pension's policy by immediately restoring the earnings link; they did raise pensions in the budget but didn't make earnings the foundation of future increases. (Castle and Townsend, 1996)

- The current level of the State Retirement Pension is too low and needs to be increased to an adequate level by a one-off topping up exercise along the lines advocated by John Smith in 1992. The government should aim to reduce means-testing rather than extend it.
- The government should ensure that everyone has an adequate minimal provision for their retirement which is sufficient to lift them out of dependency on means-tested benefits. The Conservative governments of 1979 to 1997 slashed the State Earnings Related Pension Scheme (SERPs) which had been introduced with all-party support in the 1970s. A modernised version of SERPs would be comprehensive and meet the needs of people on low incomes, unlike the stakeholder pension alternative proposed by the current government (DSS, 1998c). A return to the 'twenty best years formula' – in which the pension people receive relates to their 20 years of highest earnings – is important for manual and part-time workers and women whose

working lives are interrupted by family responsibilities and unemployment.

• Good quality occupational pensions need to be encouraged and tighter regulation of personal pensions is required to prevent misleading selling. The government proposals in the Green Paper on pensions to strengthen regulation through the Financial Services Authority are welcome. However, there are currently 22 different kinds of pension available in Britain and the Green Paper proposals will create even more schemes. There is a desperate need for legislation to help reduce the complexity of the current pensions system. Even if good financial advice was available to all, it would still be almost impossible for most people to decide which combinations they should choose among the mass of pension schemes, for example, basic state pension, the newly proposed state second pension, stakeholder pensions, defined contribution or defined benefit occupational pension (ie either final salary, group money purchase or group personal pensions), unit linked or with profits personal pensions, LISAs, SIPPs, SSASs, FURBs, etc.

Disability, long-term illness and poverty

Sick and disabled people suffer from extremely high rates of poverty and deprivation in Britain and in other countries. For example, in a statement presented to the United Nations World Summit on Social Development in 1995 on behalf of Disabled Peoples' International, Liisa Kauppinen, said:'

> We are the poorest of the poor in most societies.... Two thirds of disabled people are estimated to be without employment. Social exclusion and isolation are the day-to-day experiences of disabled people. (Kauppinen, 1995, quoted in Beresford, 1996)

Extraordinarily high levels of poverty have been recorded among disabled people in Britain in the 1980s. Berthoud et al (1993) estimated that 45% of all disabled adults were living in poverty and Gordon and Heslop (1999) estimated that 55% of disabled children and their families were living in or on the margins of poverty. Similar problems of low income and high deprivation among disabled people have also been found in Northern Ireland (Zarb and Maher, 1997).

Poverty and lack of adequate income are among the main reasons why disabled people can often become ill and why ill-health can often persist. It is self-evident that inequalities in health can be reduced if the standard of living of long-term sick and disabled people can be improved. However, welfare and benefits policy towards this group throughout much of the 20th century can best be described as 'irrational, inequitable and inadequate' and policy development was plagued by "Haphazard and piecemeal incrementalism ... when money was available or pressure strong, and have been grafted onto existing systems. Nothing has been jettisoned and nothing rethought from first principles" (Baldwin et al, 1981). The 1980s were described as "disastrous for disabled people, involving threats to opportunities, living standards, independence and choice" (Glendinning, 1991). At the end of the 1990s, the government is pledged to eliminate childhood poverty but it is silent on the poverty of elderly and disabled people. It is therefore unsurprising that analysis of government surveys has shown that 60% of disabled people have to claim 'safety net' benefits and 47% of them did not have enough to meet their minimum living costs (Berthoud et al, 1993). Independent surveys of families with disabled children have also shown that "For many, their greatest need was for more financial assistance.... Most parents felt higher weekly disability benefits would be the best way to provide further financial assistance" (Beresford, 1995).

There have been over 25 years of high quality scientific research that has consistently demonstrated that the incomes of disabled adults and children are often insufficient to meet even their basic needs (for example, see Bradshaw, 1975; Disability Alliance, 1975; Reid, 1975; Loach, 1976; Baldwin, 1977, 1985; Smyth and Robus, 1989; Glendinning, 1991; Walker et al, 1992; Berthoud et al, 1993; Beresford, 1995; Zarb and Maher, 1997; Gordon and Heslop, 1999; Kagan et al, 1998). This is a clear message that requires specific policies:

- The levels of disability benefits are too low to prevent poverty and they need to be increased, substantially in some cases, to meet the additional costs of disability and ill-health. For example, budget standards research has shown that it would cost on average £125,000 to bring up a child with a severe disability from birth to 17 years of age at 1997 prices. This is three times more than the cost of a child without a disability, if the goods and services regarded as essential were all being purchased (Dobson and Middleton, 1998). Benefits for severely disabled children would need to be increased by between 20% and 50%, depending on the child's age and type of impairment, to meet the costs of the minimum essential budgets.

- The rates of long-term disability benefits should be linked to earnings, not prices.
- There is a need for mental health component criteria to be introduced into the assessment for Disability Living Allowance (DLA). The 47-page DLA claim form needs to be simplified and proactive policies implemented to help disabled people claim all the benefits to which they are entitled.
- Any test for claimants of Incapacity Benefit must take account of fluctuating health conditions as well as the current conditions for capacity to work.
- A Disability Earnings Concession (DEC) should be introduced which allows people in receipt of disability benefits to work and earn money as and when their health allows it, without any risk to benefit entitlement. Thus, working has no effect on benefits; however, a higher tax code for DEC earners will deduct the usual tax and National Insurance, plus a reasonable percentage towards Department of Social Security, Council Tax and Housing Benefits when that person does work (DLA would be excluded from this consideration).
- The cuts in funding and eligibility criteria of the Access to Work Scheme need to be restored.
- A fully inclusive educational system is needed that delivers the same standard of education to both disabled and non-disabled children alike.

Objections to poor people getting more money

There are three types of objections that are always raised when redistributive anti-poverty policies such as those above are suggested. These are often characterised in the policy literature as (1) The 'undeserving poor' argument, (2) the argument that greater income equality is 'bad for the economy', and (3) 'the time is not yet right' argument. We will discuss these in turn.

1 'The undeserving poor'

This type of argument has a myriad of forms but generally assumes that people are not really poor because of a lack of money but because they are lazy and shiftless and/or have chosen to waste their money on drink, cigarettes, drugs or gambling. A long list of different items can be inserted here, depending upon what is considered to be reprehensible to the prevailing 'middle-class' morality of the time. The main thrust of this argument is to show that the poor are poor only because of their own fecklessness and providing them with any extra resources would only encourage them in their reprehensible ways (Gordon and Pantazis, 1997).

The attempt to divide the 'poor' into the 'deserving' (ie those who are poor through no fault of their own) and the 'undeserving', has a long history dating back at least to Elizabethan times. Indeed, it was concern about the 'residuum' (the Victorian name for the 'underclass') that resulted in the establishment of the Social Sciences in the 19th century. The residuum were the 'dangerous poor', the group of undeserving poor people who were 'criminally inclined' and detached from the values of 'right-thinking society'(Stedman-Jones, 1984). The idea of a group of criminal, feckless poor people whose pathological culture and/or genes transmitted their poverty to their children, can be traced from the Victorian residuum through theories of pauperism, social problem groups and multiple problem families to the underclass arguments of today (Macnicol, 1987; Mazumdar, 1992). The problem of poverty was blamed on 'bad' genes before the Second World War and on 'bad' culture after the discrediting of the eugenics movement by the end of the War. The underclass are currently claimed to suffer from a pathological 'culture of poverty/dependency' which causes their poverty (Bagguley and Mann, 1992).

Ideas of a 'feckless class' are unsupported by any substantial body of evidence. Despite almost 150 years of scientific investigation, often by extremely partisan investigators, not a single study has ever found any large group of people/households (ie more than 1.5% of the population) with any behaviours that could be ascribed to a culture or genetics of poverty. This failure does not result from lack of research or lack of resources. For example, the Transmitted Deprivation Programme of the 1970s lasted over 10 years, commissioned 23 empirical studies and cost over £3m at 1992 prices (Brown and Madge, 1982). The Pauper Pedigree Project of the Eugenics Society lasted over 20 years (1910–33) and the Social Survey of Merseyside Study lasted five years (Lidbetter, 1933; Caradog-Jones, 1934). The Problem Families Project started in 1947 and eventually petered out in the 1950s (Blacker, 1937, 1952). Neither these nor any other British study has ever found anything but a small number of individuals whose poverty could be ascribed to fecklessness or to 'culture/genetics of poverty/dependency'.

The 'culture of poverty/dependency' thesis requires that there is a significantly large, stable and relatively homogenous group of 'poor' people in order for a culture to develop that is different from the culture of the rest of society. The evidence we have on the prevalence and dynamics of poverty contradicts this thesis. The *Breadline Britain* survey showed that 46% of respondents have experienced at least a brief spell of living in poverty at some time in their lives and 20% of households could 'objectively' be described as 'poor'. However, only 4% of households were both currently poor and also had a long history of poverty. The experience of poverty is a widespread but, for the large majority, relatively brief phenomenon. It is, therefore, unsurprising that there is little evidence that the 'poor' have a different culture from the rest of society (Gordon and Pantazis, 1997; Gordon and Spicker, 1999). The 10-year Transmitted Deprivation Programme concluded, from a comprehensive review of the literature, that:

> Problem families do not constitute a group which is qualitatively different from families in the general population. (Rutter and Madge, 1976, p 255)

and, from the results of the 37 Transmitted Deprivation research projects, it was found that:

> All the evidence suggests that cultural values are not important for the development and transmission of deprivation. (Brown and Madge, 1982, p 226)

More recently, Bagguley and Mann (1992) commented:

> What puzzles us is why both 'left' and 'right' academics find the concept of an emergent ... underclass so attractive when it has been so thoroughly destroyed by social scientific analysis. (Bagguley and Mann, 192, p 120)

In conclusion, in the history of scientific endeavour, there cannot be many more thoroughly falsified theories than the undeserving poor argument in Britain. There is more evidence for the existence of the Loch Ness Monster than for the existence of a homogeneous group of people who form an 'underclass' in the United Kingdom. Huge amounts of money and scientific effort have been wasted over the past 150 years in unsuccessfully hunting for the undeserving poor in Britain. They simply do not exist in sufficient numbers to justify the effort or any comprehensive arguments based on their existence.

2 'It's bad for the economy'

The government's overall financial policy emphasises economic growth, and it has been argued that greater income equality is incompatible with policies that promote economic growth. However, there is evidence that the reverse is the case. As Figure 5.2 shows, economic growth and greater income equality can be mutually reinforcing, rather than incompatible.

Figure 5.2: Income inequality around 1980 and labour productivity growth from 1979 to 1990

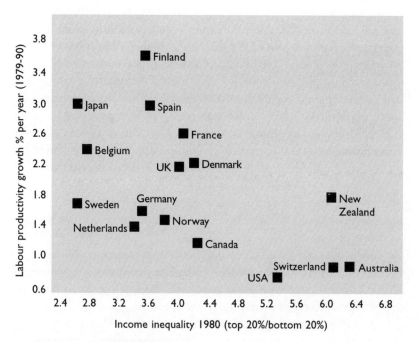

Source: Glynn and Miliband (1994)

3 'The time is not yet right'

This is a much more sophisticated objection to giving poor people more money than the rather crude 'undeserving poor' thesis. It has many forms and sophistications but the general gist is that, although it might be desirable to end poverty, it is just too risky to do anything quite so precipitous given our current state of knowledge. Without a full analysis and understanding of the recent complex structural changes in globalisation and post–Fordist capitalism (or whatever is the most popular jargon at the time), the consequences of redistribution to end poverty, however limited, might have profound, unknown and devastating repercussions which could affect us all. Giving more money to the poor could reduce our international competitiveness, put up inflation, increase dependency, lawlessness or militancy, etc. Given these threats it is probably best to do nothing and in any case things will probably get better for the 'poor' in the end given enough time.

The problem with this type of 'liberal' argument is that it is very difficult to counter as it effectively has no substance to it except the fear of the unknown. It manages to be both Distopian and Panglossian at the same time, in that it considers the current situation to be far from ideal but argues that this might still be the 'best of all possible worlds' so to attempt to change anything might be reckless and foolhardy. This is quite simply a philosophy of despair which, if accepted, would preclude any action, policy or change in any field of human existence. The argument is not based on substance and is therefore impossible to disprove. The belief that in time things will get better by themselves was eloquently demonstrated to be false by Martin Luther King while he was in prison in Birmingham, Alabama. He stated in a letter from prison that:

> Such an attitude stems from a tragic misconception of time, from the strangely irrational notion that there is something in the very flow of time that will eventually cure all ills. Actually, time itself is neutral; it can be used either destructively or constructively. More and more I feel that the people of ill will have used time much more effectively than the people of good will. We will have to repent in this generation not merely for the hateful words and actions of bad people, but for the appalling silence of good people. Human progress never rolls in on wheels of inevitability; it comes through the tireless efforts of good men willing to be co-workers with God, and without this hard work, time itself becomes an ally of the forces of social stagnation. We must use time creatively, in the knowledge that the time is always ripe to do right. (Luther King, 1965)

Conclusions

The report of the Independent Inquiry into Inequalities in Health points out, albeit in one sentence:

> We consider that without a shift of resources to the less well off, both in and out of work, little will be accomplished in terms of a reduction of health inequalities by interventions addressing particular 'downstream' influences. (1998, p 33)

Similarly, the latest World Health Organisation's annual report (WHO, 1998) states that:

> On the unfinished agenda for health, poverty remains the main item. (WHO, 1998, p 8)

Inequalities in health can only be effectively tackled by policies that reduce poverty and income inequality. The present governmental policies of assisting unemployed people to 'return to work' are helpful but not sufficient to alleviate poverty in Britain. There is also an overriding need to increase the amount of money and services received by those who cannot work.

Adequate living standards and protection against income insecurity are basic human rights enshrined in the Universal Declaration of Human Rights (Article 25) and the International Covenant on Economic, Social and Cultural Rights (Articles 7 and 9) Everybody should be entitled to a sufficient income to allow them to participate in the economic, social, cultural and political life of the country.

As we have shown throughout this book, the effects of insufficient income lead to enormous amounts of human suffering in Britain and are eventually deadly to hundreds of thousands of people. Hundreds of thousands more will die young during the first few decades of the 21st century, millions will suffer unnecessary illness and disability and tens of millions will be cheated of fair life chances for themselves and their families, until we accept that inequalities in health are the result of inequalities in income and wealth, and until those inequalities are addressed.

References

Acheson, D. (1998) 'Inequalities in health', *BMJ*, vol 317, p 1659.

Adelman, L. and Bradshaw, J. (1998) *Children in poverty in Britain: An analysis of the Family Resources Survey 1994/95*, Paper prepared as part of the ESRC project 'Poverty: the outcomes for children in the Children 5-16 Programme', York: SPRU, University of York.

Alcock, P., Craig, C., Lawless, P., Pearson, S. and Robinson, D. (1998) *Inclusive regeneration: Local authorities' corporate strategies for tackling disadvantage*, Sheffield: CRESR, Sheffield Hallam University.

Alfredsson, L., Spetz, C.L. and Theorell, T. (1985) 'Type of occupation and near-future hospitalization for myocardial infarction and some other diagnoses', *International Journal of Epidemiology*, vol 14, pp 378-88.

Arber, S. and Ginn, J. (1993) 'Gender and inequalities in health in later life', *Social Science and Medicine: Women, Men and Health Special Issue*, vol 36, no 1, pp 33-46.

Bagguley, P. and Mann, K. (1992) 'Idle thieving bastards? Scholarly representations of the underclass', *Work, Employment & Society*, vol 6, no 1, pp 113-26.

Baker, I.A., Sweetnam, P.M., Yarnell, J.W.G., Bainton, D. and Elwood, P.C. (1988) 'Haemostatic and other risk factors for ischaemic heart disease and social class: evidence from the Caerphilly and Speedwell studies', *International Journal of Epidemiology*, vol 17, pp 759-65.

Baldwin, S. (1977) *Disabled children – Counting the costs*, London: The Disability Alliance.

Baldwin, S. (1985) *The costs of caring: Families with disabled children*, London: Routledge & Kegan Paul.

Baldwin, S., Bradshaw, J., Cooke, K. and Glendinning, C. (1981) 'The disabled person and cash benefits', in D. Guthrie (ed) *Disability: Legislation and practice*, London: Macmillan.

Barker, D.J.P. (1994) *Mothers, babies and disease in later life*, London: BMJ Publications.

Barker, D.J.P. and Osmond, C. (1986) 'Childhood respiratory infection and adult chronic bronchitis in England and Wales', *BMJ*, vol 293, pp 1271-5.

Barnes, J. and Lucas, H. (1975) *Educational priority*, London: HMSO.

Bartley, M. (1994) 'Unemployment and ill health: understanding the relationship', *Journal of Epidemiology and Community Health*, vol 48, pp 333-7.

Bartley, M., Blane, D. and Montgomery, S. (1997) 'Health and the life course: why safety nets matter', *BMJ*, vol 314, pp 1194-6.

Ben-Shlomo, Y. and Chaturvedi, N. (1995) 'Assessing equity in access to health care provision in the UK: does where you live affect your chances of getting a CABG?', *Journal of Epidemiology and Community Health*, vol 49, pp 200-4.

Ben-Shlomo, Y. and Davey Smith, G. (1991) 'Deprivation in infancy or adult life: which is more important for mortality risk?', *The Lancet*, vol 337, pp 530-4.

Ben-Shlomo, Y., White, I.R. and Marmot, M. (1996) 'Does the variation in the socioeconomic characteristics of an area affect mortality?', *BMJ*, vol 312, p 1013.

Benzeval, M., Judge, K. and Whitehead, M. (1995) *Tackling inequalities in health*, London: The King's Fund.

Beresford, B. (1995) *Expert opinions: A national survey of parents caring for a severely disabled child*, Bristol: The Policy Press.

Beresford, P. (1996) 'Poverty and disabled people: challenging dominant debates and policies', *Disability and Society*, vol 11, no 4, pp 553-67.

Berthoud, R., Lakey, J. and McKay S. (1993) *The economic problems of disabled people*, London: Policy Studies Institute.

Bethune, A. (1997) 'Unemployment and mortality', in F. Drever and M. Whitehead (eds) *Health inequalities*, ONS, Series DS No 15, London: The Stationery Office.

Betts, G. (1993) *Local government and inequalities in health*, Aldershot: Avebury.

Bines, W. (1994) *The health of single homeless people*, York: Centre for Housing Policy, University of York.

Black, D., Morris, J.N., Smith, C. and Townsend, P. (1999) 'Better benefits for health: plan to implement the central recommendations of the Acheson report', *BMJ*, vol 318, pp 724-7.

Blackburn, C. (1991) *Poverty and health: Working with families*, Milton Keynes: Open University Press.

Blacker, C.P. (1937) *A social problem group?*, London: Oxford University Press.

Blacker, C.P. (ed) (1952) *Problem families: Five enquiries*, London: Eugenics Society.

Blair, T. (1999) Beveridge Lecture at Toynbee Hall, London on 18 March, London: Cabinet Office.

Blane, D. (1985) 'An assessment of the Black Report's "explanations of health inequalities"', *Sociology of Health and Illness*, vol 7, pp 423-45.

Blane, D. and Drever, F. (1998) 'Inequality among men in standardised years of potential life lost, 1970-73', *BMJ*, vol 317, p 255.

Blane, D., Bartley, M. and Davey Smith, G. (1997) 'Disease aetiology and materialist explanations of socioeconomic mortality differentials', *European Journal of Public Health*, vol 7, pp 385-91.

Blane, D., Bartley, M. and Davey Smith, G. (1998) 'Disease aetiology and materialist explanations of socioeconomic mortality differentials: a research note', *European Journal of Public Health*, vol 8, no 3, pp 259-60.

Blane, D., Davey Smith, G. and Bartley, M. (1993) 'Social selection: what does it contribute to social class differences in health?', *Sociology of Health and Illness*, vol 15, no 1, pp 1-15.

Blaxter, M. (1991) 'Fifty years on – inequalities in health', in M. Murphy and J. Hobcraft (eds) *Population research in Britain: A supplement to Population Studies*, vol 45, Cambridge: Cambridge University Press.

Bloor, M., Samphier, M. and Prior, L. (1987) 'Artefact explanations of inequalities in health: an assessment of the evidence', *Sociology of Health and Illness*, vol 9, pp 231-64.

Braddon, F.E.M., Wadsworth, M.E.J., Davies, J.M.C. and Cripps, H.A. (1988) 'Social and regional differences in food and alcohol consumption and their measurement in a national birth cohort', *Journal of Epidemiology and Community Health*, vol 42, pp 341-9.

Bradshaw, J. (1975) *The financial needs of disabled children*, London: The Disability Alliance.

Bradshaw, J. (ed) (1993) *Budget standards for the United Kingdom*, Aldershot: Avebury.

Bradshaw, J. (1998) 'The prevalence of child poverty in the UK: a comparative analysis', Children and Social Exclusion Conference, University of Hull.

Bradshaw, J. and Barnes, H. (1999: forthcoming) 'Relating inputs to outcomes: child poverty and family transfers in comparative perspective', in H. Emanuel (ed) *Issues in social security*, Aldershot: Ashgate.

Bradshaw, J. and Chen, J.-R. (1997) 'Poverty in the UK: a comparison with nineteen other countries', *Benefits*, vol 18, pp 13-17.

Bramley, G. (1990) 'The demand for local government services: survey evidence on usage, distribution and externalities', *Local Government Studies*, November/December, pp 35-61.

Bramley, G. (1997) 'Poverty and local public services', in D. Gordon and C. Pantazis (eds) *Breadline Britain in the 1990s*, Aldershot: Ashgate.

Bramley, G. and Le Grand, J. (1992) *Who uses local services? Striving for equity*, The Belgrave Papers No 4, London and Luton: Local Government Management Board.

Bramley, G. and Smart, G. (1993) *Who benefits from local services? Comparative evidence from different local authorities*, Welfare State Programme Discussion Paper WSP/91, Suntory-Toyota International Centre for Economics and Related Disciplines, London: London School of Economics.

Bramley, G., Le Grand, J. and Low, W. (1989) 'How far is the poll tax a "community charge"? The implications of service usage evidence', *Policy & Politics*, vol 17, no 3, pp 187-205.

Brimblecombe, N., Dorling, D. and Shaw, M. (1999) 'Mortality and migration in Britain, first results from the British Household Panel Survey', *Social Science and Medicine*, vol 49, pp 981-8.

Brittan, S. and Webb, S. (1990) *Beyond the welfare state: An examination of basic incomes in a market economy*, The David Hume Institute, Aberdeen: Aberdeen University Press.

Brown, G. and Cook, R. (eds) (1983) *Scotland: The real divide: Poverty and deprivation in Scotland*, Edinburgh: Mainstream Publishing.

Brown, M. and Madge, N. (1982) *Despite the welfare state: A report on the SSRC/DHSS Programme of Research into Transmitted Deprivation*, SSRC/DHSS Studies in Deprivation and Disadvantage, London: Heinemann Educational Books.

Bunting, J. (1997) 'Appendix A: sources and methods', in F. Drever and M. Whitehead (eds) *Health inequalities: Decennial supplement*, ONS, London: The Stationery Office.

Buring, J.E., Evans, D.A., Fiore, M., Rosner, B. and Hennekens, C.H. (1987) 'Occupation and risk of death from coronary heart disease', *JAMA*, vol 258, pp 791-2.

Burke, K. (1999) 'Doctors fear that inequalities are slipping down the agenda', *BMJ*, vol 319, p 144.

Cade, J.E., Barker, D.J.P., Margetts, B.M. and Morris, J.A. (1988) 'Diet and inequalities in health in three English towns', *BMJ*, vol 296, pp 1359-62.

Calman, K. (1998) *On the state of the public health 1997: The annual report of the Chief Medical Officer of the Department of Health for the year 1997*, London: The Stationery Office.

Caradog Jones, D. (ed) (1934) *The social survey of Merseyside, Vol III*, London: Hodder & Stoughton.

Carstairs, V. (1994) 'Health care needs, deprivation, and the resource allocation formula', in E. Gilman, S. Munday, L. Somervaille and R. Strachan (eds) *Resource allocation and health needs: From research to policy*, London: HMSO.

Carstairs, V. and Morris, R. (1989a) 'Deprivation: explaining differences in mortality between Scotland and England and Wales', *BMJ*, vol 299, pp 886-9.

Carstairs, V. and Morris, R. (1989b) 'Deprivation and mortality: an alternative to social class?', *Community Medicine*, vol 11, pp 210-19.

Castle, B. and Townsend, P (1996) *We can afford the welfare state*, London: T&G.

Castle, B., Davies, B., Land, H., Townsend, P., Lynes, T. and Macintyre, K. (1998) *Fair shares for pensioners: Evidence to the Pensions Review Body*, London: Security in Retirement for Everyone.

CDP (Community Development Project) (1977) *Gilding the ghetto: The state and the poverty experiments*, Nottingham: CDP and The Russell Press Limited.

Chadwick, E. (1842) *Report on the sanitary condition of the labouring population of Great Britain*, London: HMSO.

Chadwick, M., O'Donoghue, C., Redmond, G. and Sutherland, H. (1997) *Neither Santa Claus nor Scrooge?*, Microsimulation Research Unit Note, DAE, Cambridge: University of Cambridge.

Charlton, J. (1997) 'Trends in all-cause mortality: 1841-1994', in J. Charlton and M. Murphy (eds) *The health of adult Britain, 1841-1994, Volume 1*, London: The Stationery Office.

Charlton, J. and Murphy, M. (eds) (1997) *The health of adult Britain 1841-1994*, London: The Stationery Office.

Chaturvedi, N. and Ben Shlomo, Y. (1995) 'From surgery to surgeon: does deprivation influence access to care?', *British Journal of General Practice*, vol 45, pp 127-31.

Chaturvedi, N., Rai, J. and Ben Shlomo, Y. (1997) 'Lay diagnosis and health care seeking behaviour for chest pain in South Asians and Europeans', *The Lancet*, vol 350, pp 1578-83.

Church, J. and Whyman, S. (1997) 'A review of recent social trends and economic trends', in F. Drever and M. Whitehead (eds) *Health inequalities: Decennial supplement*, ONS, London: The Stationery Office.

Clarke, T. and McCrae, J. (1998) *Taxing Child Benefit*, Commentary 74, London: Institute for Fiscal Studies, December.

Coggon, D., Osmond, C. and Barker, D.J.P. (1990) 'Stomach cancer and migration within England and Wales', *British Journal of Cancer*, vol 61, pp 573-4.

Cohen, R., Coxall, J., Craig, G. and Sadiq-Sangster, A.S. (1992) *Hardship in Britain: Being poor in the 1990s*, London: Child Poverty Action Group.

Congdon, P. (1995) 'The impact of area context on long term illness and premature mortality: an illustration of multi-level analysis', *Regional Studies*, vol 29, no 4, pp 327-44.

Cordon, A. (1995) *New perspectives on take-up: A literature review*, London: HMSO.

Dale, A. and Marsh, C. (eds) (1993) *The 1991 Census user's guide*, London: HMSO.

Davey Smith, G. and Ben-Shlomo, Y. (1997) 'Geographical and social class differences in stroke mortality – the influence of early-life factors', *Journal of Epidemiology and Community Health*, vol 51, pp 134-7.

Davey Smith, G. and Dorling, D. (1996) ' "I'm all right John": voting patterns and mortality in England and Wales, 1981-92', *BMJ*, vol 313, pp 1573-7.

Davey Smith, G. and Gordon, D. (2000: forthcoming) 'Poverty across the lifecourse and health', in C. Pantazis and D. Gordon (eds) *Tackling inequalities: Where are we now and what can be done?*, Bristol: The Policy Press.

Davey Smith, G. and Hart, C. (1998) 'Socioeconomic factors and determinants of mortality', *JAMA*, vol 280, no 20, pp 1744-5.

Davey Smith, G. and Phillips, A.N. (1990) 'Declaring independence: why we should be cautious', *Journal of Epidemiology and Community Health*, vol 44, pp 257-8.

Davey Smith, G., Bartley, M. and Blane, D. (1990b) 'The Black Report on socioeconomic inequalities in health 10 years on', *BMJ*, vol 301, pp 373-7.

Davey Smith, G., Blane, D. and Bartley, M. (1994) 'Explanations for socio-economic differentials in mortality: evidence from Britain and elsewhere', *European Journal of Public Health*, vol 4, pp 131-44.

Davey Smith, G., Morris, J.N. and Shaw, M. (1998a) 'The independent inquiry into inequalities in health', *BMJ*, vol 317, pp 1465-6.

Davey Smith, G., Shaw, M. and Dorling, D. (1998e) 'Shrinking areas and mortality', *The Lancet*, vol 352, pp 1139-40.

Davey Smith, G., Shipley, M.J. and Rose, G. (1990a) 'The magnitude and causes of socio-economic differentials in mortality: further evidence from the Whitehall study', *Journal of Epidemiology Community Health*, vol 44, pp 265-70.

Davey Smith, G., Hart, C., Blane, D. and Hole, D. (1998c) 'Adverse socioeconomic conditions in childhood and cause-specific adult mortality: prospective observational study', *BMJ*, vol 316, pp 1631-5.

Davey Smith, G., Leon, D., Shipley, M.J. and Rose, G. (1991) 'Socioeconomic differentials in cancer among men', *International Journal of Epidemiology*, vol 30, pp 339-45.

Davey Smith, G., Hart, C., Blane, D., Gillis, C. and Hawthorne, V. (1997) 'Lifetime socioeconomic position and mortality: prospective observational study', *BMJ*, vol 314, pp 547-52.

Davey Smith, G., Hart, C., Watt, G., Hole, D. and Hawthorne, V. (1998d) 'Individual social class, area-based deprivation, cardiovascular disease risk factors, and mortality: the Renfrew and Paisley study', *Journal of Epidemiology and Community Health*, vol 52, pp 399-405.

Davey Smith, G., Neaton, J.D., Wentworth, D., Stamler, R. and Stamler, J. (1996a) 'Socioeconomic differentials in mortality risk among men screened for the Multiple Risk Factor Intervention Trial: Part I – results for 300,685 white men', *American Journal of Public Health*, vol 86, pp 486-96.

Davey Smith, G., Neaton, J.D., Wentworth, D., Stamler, R. and Stamler, J. (1996b) 'Socioeconomic differentials in mortality risk among men screened for the Multiple Risk Factor Intervention Trial: Part II – results for 20,224 black men', *American Journal of Public Health*, vol 86, pp 497-504.

Davey Smith, G., Hart, C., Hole, D., MacKinnon, P., Gillis, C., Watt, G., Blane, D. and Hawthorne, V. (1998b) 'Education and occupational social class: which is the more important indicator of mortality risk?', *Journal of Epidemiology and Community Health*, vol 52, pp 153-60.

Denham, J. and DoH (Department of Health) (1999) 'Health Action Zones invited to apply for £4.5m funding for innovation and fellowship', Press Release 1999/0386, Friday 25 June.

Desai, M. (1998) 'A basic income proposal', in R. Skidelsky, W. Eltis, E. Davis, N. Gemmell and M. Desai (eds) *The state of the future*, London: Social Market Foundation.

DHSS (Department of Health and Social Security) (1980) *Inequalities in health: Report of a working group*, London: DHSS (Black Report).

Dilnot, A. (1998) *Evidence to Social Security Committee*, 16 December.

Disability Alliance, The (1975) *Poverty and disability: The case for a comprehensive income scheme for disabled people*, London: The Disability Alliance.

Dobson, F. and DoH (Department of Health) (1997a) 'Government takes action to reduce health inequalities', Press release in response to the Joseph Rowntree Publication *Death in Britain*, DoH Press Release 97/192, 11 August.

Dobson, F. and DoH (1997b) 'Healthy homes for healthy lives, Frank Dobson addresses National Housing Federation', DoH Press Release 97/282, 16 October.

Dobson, F and DoH (1997c) 'Partnership is the key to improving public health', DoH Press Release 97/365, 28 November.

Dobson, F. and DoH (1998a) 'The whole of the government tackling health inequalities – a new spirit of optimism and hope' says Frank Dobson, DoH Press Release 98/018, 15 January.

Dobson, F. and DoH (1998b) 'Government committed to greatest ever reduction in health inequalities' says Frank Dobson, Acheson Report into Inequalities in Health welcomed, DoH Press Release 98/0547, 26 November.

Dobson, B. and Middleton, S. (1998) *Paying to care: The cost of childhood disability*, York: York Publishing Services.

DoH (Department of Health) (1996) *Low income, food, nutrition and health: Strategies for improvement*, London: DoH.

DoH (1997) *The new NHS – Modern and dependable*, London: The Stationery Office.

DoH (1998a) *Our Healthier Nation: A new contract for health*, London: The Stationery Office.

DoH (1998b) 'Frank Dobson gives the go-ahead for first wave of health action zones', Press Release 98/120, Tuesday 31 March.

DoH (1999a) *Saving lives: Our healthier nation*, London: The Stationery Office.

DoH (1999b) 'Seven million people to benefit from fifteen new Health Action Zones', Press Release 1999/0259, Friday 23 April.

DoH (1999c) *Reducing health inequalities:An action report*, London: DoH.

Dorling, D. (1995) *A new social atlas of Britain*, Chichester:Wiley.

Dorling, D. (1997) *Death in Britain: How local mortality rates have changed: 1950s-1990s*, York: Joseph Rowntree Foundation.

Dowler, E. (1996) 'Women and food in poor families: focus for concern?', in J. Butriss and K. Hyman (eds) *Focus on women: Nutrition and health*, London: National Dairy Council, pp 69-81.

Dowler, E. and Calvert, C. (1995) *Nutrition and diet in lone-parent households in London*, London: Family Policy Studies Centre.

Drever, F. (1997) 'Appendix B', in F. Drever and M. Whitehead (eds) *Health inequalities*, London:The Stationery Office.

Drever, F. and Bunting, J. (1997) 'Patterns and trends in male mortality', in F. Drever and M. Whitehead (eds) *Health inequalities*, London: The Stationery Office.

Drever, F. and Whitehead, M. (1997) (eds) *Health inequalities,* London: The Stationery Office.

DSS (1996) *Households Below Average Income*, London: The Stationery Office.

DSS (1997) *Households Below Average Income*, London: The Stationery Office.

DSS (Department of Social Security) (1998a) (annual) *Households Below Average Income 1979-1996/7*, London:The Stationery Office.

DSS (1998b) *New ambitions for our country:A new contract for welfare*, London: The Stationery Office.

DSS (1998c) *A new contract for welfare: Partnership in pensions*, Cmd 4179, London:The Stationery Office.

Eachus, J., Williams, M., Chan, P., Davey Smith, G., Grainge, M., Donovan, J. and Frankel, S. (1996) 'Deprivation and cause specific morbidity: evidence from the Somerset and Avon survey of health', *BMJ*, vol 312, pp 287-92.

Ecob, R. and Davey Smith, G. (1999) 'Income and health: what is the nature of the relationship?', *Social Science & Medicine*, vol 48, no 5, pp 693-705.

Ellaway, A. and Macintyre, S. (1996) 'Does where you live predict health related behaviours? A case study in Glasgow', *Health Bulletin (Edinburgh)*, vol 54, pp 443-6.

Ellaway, A., Anderson, A. and Macintyre, S. (1997) 'Does area of residence affect body size and shape?', *International Journal of Obesity*, vol 21, pp 304-8.

Eurobarometer (1989) Special issue on racism and xenophobia, *Eurobarometer*, November, pp 1-5.

Eurostat (1994) European Household Community Panel Survey.

Erren, T.C., Jacobsen, M. and Piekarski, C. (1999) 'Synergy between asbestos and smoking on lung cancer risks', *Epidemiology*, vol 10, pp 405-11.

Fehily, A.M., Phillips, K.M. and Yarnell, J.W.G. (1984) 'Diet, smoking, social class, and body mass index in the Caerphilly Heart Disease study', *American Journal of Clinical Nutrition*, vol 40, pp 827-33.

Ferrie, J., Shipley, M.J., Marmot, M.G., Stansfeld, S. and Davey Smith, G. (1995) 'Health effects of anticipation of job change and non-employment: longitudinal data from the Whitehall II study', *BMJ*, vol 311, pp 1265-9.

Ferrie, J., Shipley M.J., Marmot, M.G., Stansfeld, S. and Davey Smith, G. (1998) 'An uncertain future: the health effects of threats to employment security in white-collar men and women', *American Journal of Public Health*, vol 88, pp 1031-6.

Filakti, H. and Fox, J. (1995) 'Differences in mortality by housing tenure and by car access from the OPCS Longitudinal Study', *Population Trends*, vol 81, pp 27-30.

Fisher, K. and Collins, J. (1993) 'Access to health care', in K. Fisher and J. Collins (eds) *Homelessness, health care and welfare provision*, London: Routledge, pp 32-50.

Forsdahl, A. (1977) 'Are poor living conditions in childhood and adolescence an important risk factor for arteriosclerotic heart disease', *British Journal of Preventive and Social Medicine*, vol 31, pp 91-5.

Forsdahl, A. (1978) 'Living conditions in childhood and subsequent development of risk factors for arteriosclerotic heart disease. The cardiovascular survey in Finnmark 1974-7', *Journal of Epidemiology and Community Health*, vol 32, pp 34-7.

Frankel, S., Elwood, P., Sweetnam, P., Yarnell, J. and Davey Smith, G. (1996) 'Birthweight, body mass index in middle age, and incident coronary heart disease', *The Lancet*, vol 348, pp 1478-80.

Fuchs, V.R. (1979) 'Economics, health, and post-industrial society', *Millbank Memorial Fund Quarterly*, vol 57, pp 153-82.

GHS (General Household Survey) (1996) *Living in Britain*, ONS, London: The Stationery Office.

Glendinning, C. (1991) 'Losing ground: social policy and disabled people in Great Britain 1980-1990', *Disability, Handicap & Society*, vol 6, no 1, pp 3-19.

Glennerster, H., Lupton, R., Noden, P. and Power, A. (1999) *Poverty, social exclusion and neighbourhood: Studying the area bases of social exclusion*, CASE Paper 22, London: London School of Economics.

Glynn, A. and Miliband, D. (1994) *Paying for inequality: The economic costs of social injustice*, London: Rivers Oran Press.

Goddard, M. and Smith, P. (1998) *Equity of access to health care*, York: University of York.

Goldblatt, P. (1990a) 'Social class mortality differences', in N.M. Mascie-Taylor (ed) *The biology of social class*, Oxford: Oxford University Press.

Goldblatt, P. (1990b) 'Mortality and alternative social classifications', in P. Goldblatt (ed) *Longitudinal Study. Mortality and social organisation 1971-1981*, OPCS, London: HMSO, pp 164-90.

Goodman, A. and Webb, S. (1995) *The distribution of UK household expenditure, 1979-92*, London: Institute for Fiscal Studies.

Gordon, D. (1995) 'Census based deprivation indices: their weighting and validation', *Journal of Epidemiology and Community Health*, vol 49(Supplement 2), pp 39-44.

Gordon, D. and Forrest, R. (1995) *People and places Volume II: Social and economic distinctions in England – A 1991 Census Atlas*, Bristol: SAUS Publications.

Gordon, D. and Heslop, P. (1999) 'Poverty and disabled children', in D. Dorling and S. Simpson (eds) *Statistics in society: The arithmetic of politics*, London: Arnold.

Gordon, D. and Loughran, F. (1997) 'Child poverty and needs based budget allocation', *Research, Policy and Planning,* vol 15, no 3, pp 28-38.

Gordon, D. and Pantazis, C. (eds) (1997) *Breadline Britain in the 1990s*, Aldershot: Ashgate.

Gordon, D. and Spicker, P. (eds) (1999) *The international glossary on poverty*, New York and London: Zed Books.

Gordon, D., Shaw, M., Dorling, D. and Davey Smith, G. (1999) *Inequalities in health: The evidence*, Bristol: The Policy Press.

Graham, H. (1995) 'Cigarette smoking: a light on gender and class inequality in Britain?', *Journal of Social Policy*, vol 24, no 4, pp 509-27.

Graham, H. (1996) 'The health experiences of mothers and young children on income support', *Benefits*, September/October, pp 10-13.

Gregg, P. and Wadsworth, J. (1996) 'More work in fewer households?', in J. Hills (ed) *New inequalities: The changing distribution of income and wealth in the United Kingdom*, Cambridge: Cambridge University Press

Gregory, J., Foster, K., Tyler, H. and Wiseman, M. (1990) *The dietary and nutritional survey of British adults*, London: HMSO.

Haan, M.N., Kaplan, G.A. and Camacho, T. (1987) 'Poverty and health: prospective evidence from the Alameda County study', *American Journal of Epidemiology*, vol 125, pp 989-98.

Haan, M.N., Kaplan, G.A. and Syme, S.L. (1989) 'Socioeconomic status and health: old observations and new thoughts', in J.P. Bunker, D.S. Gomby and B.H. Kehrer (eds) *Pathways to health: The role of social factors*, Menlo Park, CA: The Henry J. Kaiser Family Foundation, pp 76-135.

Hansbro, J., Bridgwood, A., Morgan A. and Hickman, M. (1997) 'Health in England: what people know, what people think, what people do', ONS, London: The Stationery Office.

Hansson, L.-E., Bergström, R., Sparén, P. and Adami, H.-O. (1991) 'The decline in the incidence of stomach cancer in Sweden 1960-1984: a birth cohort phenomenon', *International Journal of Cancer*, vol 47, pp 499-503.

Hart, C.L., Davey Smith, G. and Blane, D. (1998) 'Social mobility and 21-year mortality in a cohort of Scottish men', *Social Science and Medicine*, vol 47, pp 1121-30.

Hattersley, L. (1999) 'Trends in life expectancy by social class – an update', *Health Statistics Quarterly*, vol 2, pp 16-24.

Heath, A.F. and Clifford, P. (1990) 'Class inequalities in education in the twentieth century', *Journal of the Royal Statistical Society A*, vol 153, pp 1-16.

HEFCE (Higher Education Funding Council for England) (1997) *The influence of neighbourhood type on participation in higher education*, Bristol: HEFCE.

Hein, H.O., Suadicani, P. and Gyntelberg, F. (1992) 'Ischaemic heart disease incidence by social class and form of smoking: the Copenhagen male study – 17 years' follow-up', *Journal of Internal Medicine*, vol 231, pp 477-83.

Hertz-Picciotto, I., Smith, A.H., Holtzman, D., Lipsett, M. and Alexeeff, G. (1992) 'Synergism between occupational arsenic exposure and smoking in the induction of lung cancer', *Epidemiology*, vol 3, no 1, pp 23-31.

Higgens, J. (1998) 'HAZs Warning', *Health Service Journal*, 16 April, pp 24-5.

Hills, J. (1995) *Income and wealth, vol 2*, York: Joseph Rowntree Foundation.

Hills, J. (1998) *Income and wealth: The latest evidence*, York: Joseph Rowntree Foundation.

Holme, I., Helgeland. A., Hjermann, I., Leren, P. and Lund-Larsen, P.G. (1981) 'Physical activity at work and at leisure in relation to coronary risk factors and social class', *Acta Med Scand*, vol 209, pp 277-83.

Howarth, C., Kenway, P., Palmer, G. and Street, C. (1998) *Monitoring poverty and social exclusion: Labour's inheritance*, York: Joseph Rowntree Foundation.

Hunter, D. (1955) *The diseases of occupations*, London: Hodder & Stoughton.

Immervoll, H., Mitton, L., O'Donoghue, C. and Sutherland, H. (1999) *Budgeting for fairness? The distributional effects of three Labour budgets*, Microsimulation Research Unit Note MU/RN/32, DAE, Cambridge: University of Cambridge.

Independent Inquiry into Inequalities in Health (1998) London: The Stationery Office.

Jones, G. (1999) 'Labour "putting profit before redistribution"', *The Daily Telegraph*, 3 February.

Jones, K. and Duncan, C. (1995) 'Individuals and their ecologies: analysing the geography of chronic illness within a multilevel modelling framework', *Health and Place*, vol 1, no 1, pp 27-40.

Jowell, R. (ed) (1991-98) *British Social Attitudes, 8th to 15th Reports*, London: SCPR.

Jowell, T. and DoH (Department of Health) (1997a) 'New mission to tackle inequalities that lead to ill health – Tessa Jowell', Press release of first major speech at Royal College of Midwives Annual Conference, DoH Press Release 97/095, 15 May.

Jowell, T. and DoH (1997b) 'Tessa Jowell pledges action to tackle health divide', Press release welcoming the publication of the ONS Decennial Supplement on *Health inequalities*, DoH Press Release 97/214, 8 September.

Jowell, T. and DoH (1997c) 'Action for health – the ultimate partnership scheme', DoH Press Release 97/309, 29 October.

Jowell, T. and DoH (1998a) 'Minister pledges action to tackle health inequalities for lone parents and their children', DoH Press Release 98/023, 21 January.

Jowell, T. and DoH (1998b) *'Our Healthier Nation* – publication of Green Paper on public health', DoH Press Release 98/050, 5 February.

Kagan, C., Lewis, S. and Heaton, P. (1998) *Accounts of working parents of disabled children*, London: Family Policy Studies Centre (in association with the Joseph Rowntree Foundation).

Kaplan, G.A. and Salonen, J.T. (1990) 'Socioeconomic conditions in childhood and ischaemic heart disease during middle age', *BMJ*, vol 301, pp 1121-3.

Kaplan, G.A., Pamuk, E.R., Lynch, J.W., Cohen, R. and Balfour, J. (1996) 'Inequality in income and mortality in the United States: analysis of mortality and potential pathways', *BMJ*, vol 312, pp 999-1003.

Karasek, R., Baker, D., Marxer, F., Ahlbom, A. and Theorell, T. (1981) 'Job decision latitude, job demands and cardiovascular disease: a prospective study of Swedish men', *American Journal of Public Health*, vol 71, pp 694-705.

Kempson, E. (1996) *Life on a low income*, York: Joseph Rowntree Foundation.

Kenkel, D.S. (1991) 'Health behavior, health knowledge, and schooling', *Journal of Political Economy*, vol 99, pp 287-305.

Kennedy, B.P., Kawachi, I. and Prothrow-Stith, D. (1996) 'Income distribution and mortality: cross sectional ecological study of the Robin Hood index in the United States', *BMJ*, vol 312, pp 1004-7.

Krieger, N. and Fee, E. (1994) 'Social class: the missing link in US health data', *International Journal of Health Services*, vol 24, pp 25-44.

Kuh, D. and Ben-Shlomo, Y. (eds) (1997) *A life course approach to chronic disease epidemiology*, Oxford: Oxford Medical Publications.

Last, J. (1995) *A dictionary of epidemiology*, Oxford: Oxford University Press.

Lee, P., Murie, A. and Gordon, D. (1995) *Area measures of deprivation*, Birmingham: CURS, University of Birmingham.

Leon, D.A., Koupilova, I. and Lithell, H.O., Berglund, L., Mohsen, R., Vagero, D., Lithell, U.-B. and McKeigue, P. (1996) 'Failure to realise growth potential in utero and adult obesity in relation to blood pressure in 50 year old Swedish men', *BMJ*, vol 312, pp 401-6.

Lewis, G. and Sloggett, A. (1998) 'Suicide, deprivation, and unemployment: record linkage study', *BMJ*, vol 317, pp 1283-6.

Lewis, G., Bebbington, P., Brugha, T., Farrell, M., Gill, B., Jenkins, R. and Meltzer, H. (1998) 'Socioeconomic status, standard of living, and neurotic disorder', *The Lancet*, vol 352, pp 605-9.

Lidbetter, E.J. (1933) *Heredity and the social problem group, Vol 1*, London: Edward Arnold.

Lithell, H.O., McKeigue, P.M., Berglund, L., Mohsen, R., Lithell, U.-B. and Leon, D.A. (1996) 'Relation of size at birth to non-insulin dependent diabetes and insulin concentrations in men aged 50-60 years', *BMJ*, vol 312, pp 406-10.

Loach, I. (1976) *The price of deafness: A review of the financial and employment problems of the deaf and hard of hearing*, London: The Disability Alliance.

Lobstein, T. (1995) 'The increasing cost of a healthy diet', *Food Magazine*, vol 31, p 17.

Lowry, S. (1989) 'Housing and health: temperature and humidity', *BMJ*, vol 299, pp 1326-8.

Luther King, M. (1965) *Why we can't wait*, London: Harper & Row Ltd.

Lynch, J.W. and Kaplan, G.A. (1997) 'Understanding how inequality in the distribution of income affects health', *Journal of Health Psychology*, vol 2, no 3, pp 297-314.

McCarthy, P., Byrne, D., Harrison, S. and Keighley, J. (1985) 'Respiratory conditions: effect of housing and other factors', *Journal of Epidemiology and Community Health*, vol 39, pp 15-19.

MacFarlane, A. and Mugford, M. (1984) 'Characteristics of parents and the circumstances in which they live', in A. MacFarlane and M. Mugford, *Birth counts: Statistics of pregnancy and childbirth*, London: HMSO.

Macintyre, S. (1997) 'The Black Report and beyond: what are the issues?', *Social Science and Medicine*, vol 44, no 6, pp 723-45.

Macintyre, S., MacIver, S. and Sooman, A. (1993) 'Area, class and health: should we be focusing on places or people?', *Journal of Social Policy*, vol 22, no 2, pp 213-34.

Macnicol, J. (1987) 'In pursuit of the underclass', *Journal of Social Policy*, vol 16, no 3, pp 293-318.

Majeed, A., Chaturvedi, N., Reading, R. and Ben Shlomo, Y. (1994) 'Monitoring and promoting equity in primary and acute care', *BMJ*, vol 308, p 1426.

Mann, S.L., Wadsworth, M.E.J. and Colley, J.R.T. (1992) 'Accumulation of factors influencing respiratory illness in members of a national birth cohort and their offspring', *Journal of Epidemiology and Community Health*, vol 46, pp 286-92.

Mare, R.D. (1990) 'Socioeconomic careers and differential mortality among older men in the United States', in J.Vallin, S. D' Souza and A. Palloni (eds) *Measurement and analysis of mortality: New approaches*, Oxford: Clarendon Press, pp 362-87.

Marmot, M.G. and Theorell, T. (1989) 'Social class and cardiovascular disease: the contribution of work', *International Journal of Health Services*, vol 18, pp 659-74.

Marmot, M.G., Bobak, M. and Davey Smith, G. (1995) 'Explanations for social inequalities in health', in B.C. Amick, S. Levine, A. Tarlov and D.C. Walsh (eds) *Society and health*, Oxford: Oxford University Press.

Marmot, M.G., Shipley, M.J. and Rose, G. (1984) 'Inequalities in death – specific explanations of a general pattern?', *The Lancet*, vol 1, pp 1003-6.

Marmot, M.G., Rose, G., Shipley, M. and Hamilton, P.J.S. (1978) 'Employment grade and coronary heart disease in British civil servants', *Journal of Epidemiology and Community Health*, vol 32, pp 244-9.

Martin, C.J., Platt, S.D. and Hunt, S. (1987) 'Housing conditions and health', *BMJ*, vol 294, pp 1125-7.

Mazumdar, P.M.H. (1992) *Eugenics, human genetics and human failings*, London and New York: Routledge.

Mendall, M.A., Goggin, P.M. and Molineaux, N. (1992) 'Childhood living conditions and *Helicobacter pylori* seropositivity in adult life', *The Lancet*, vol 339, pp 896-7.

M'Gonigle, G.C.M. and Kirby, J. (1936) *Poverty and public health*, London: Victor Gollancz Ltd.

Middleton, S., Ashworth, K. and Braithwaite, I. (1996) *Small fortunes: Spending on children, childhood poverty and parental sacrifice*, York: Joseph Rowntree Foundation.

Milburn, A. and DoH (1997) '£30 million for new partnerships to target health inequalities – Invitations for participation in Health Action Zones announced', DoH Press Release 97/312, 30 October.

Milton Keynes Council (1999) Milton Keynes Council Meeting Minutes, Budget Referendum Results, 2 March, p 6.

Montgomery, S., Cook, D., Bartley, M. and Wadsworth, M. (1999) 'Unemployment pre-dates symptoms of depression and anxiety resulting in medical consultation in young men', *International Journal of Epidemiology*, vol 28, pp 95-100.

Morgan, M., Heller, R.F. and Swerdlow, A. (1989) 'Changes in diet and coronary heart disease mortality among social classes in Great Britain', *Journal of Epidemiology and Community Health*, vol 43, pp 162-7.

Morris, J.K., Cook, D.G. and Shaper, A.G. (1994) 'Loss of employment and mortality', *BMJ*, vol 308, pp 1135-9.

Moser, K., Goldblatt. P., Fox, J. and Jones, D. (1990) 'Unemployment and mortality', in P. Goldblatt (ed) *Longitudinal Study: Mortality and social organisation*, London: HMSO, pp 81-97.

Najman, J.M. (1980) 'Theories of disease causation and the concept of general susceptibility: a review', *Social Science and Medicine*, vol 14a, pp 231-7.

Najman, J.M. (1993) 'Health and poverty: past, present and prospects for the future', *Social Science and Medicine*, vol 36, no 2, pp 157-66.

Najman, J.M. and Congalton, A.A. (1979) 'Australian occupational mortality, 1965-1967: cause specific or general susceptibility?', *Sociology of Health and Illness*, vol 1, pp 158-76.

NCH Action for Children (1995) *Factfile '95*, Rochester: NCH Action for Children.

NCH Action for Children (1998) *Factfile '99*, Rochester: NCH Action for Children.

New Earnings survey (1991) Department of Employment, London: HMSO.

Oldfield, N. and Yu, A.C.S. (1993) *The cost of a child: Living standards for the 1990s*, London: Child Poverty Action Group.

ONS (Office for National Statistics) (1996) *Mortality statistics: Childhood, infant and perinatal 1993 and 1994*, Series DH3 no 27, London: The Stationery Office.

ONS (1997) *Mortality statistics: Childhood, infant and perinatal 1995*, Series DH3 no 28, London: The Stationery Office.

ONS (1998a) *Family spending*, Report of the Family Expenditure Survey, London: The Stationery Office.

ONS (1998b) *Mortality statistics: Childhood, infant and perinatal 1996*, Series DH3 no 29, London: The Stationery Office.

Oorschot, W. (1995) 'Take it or leave it: a study of non-take-up of social security benefits', PhD Thesis, Tilburg University.

OPCS (Office of Population Censuses and Surveys) (1978) *Occupational mortality 1970-1972*, London: HMSO.

Pamuk, E.R. (1985) 'Social class inequality in mortality from 1921 to 1972 in England and Wales', *Population Studies*, vol 39, pp 17-31.

Pantazis, C. and Gordon, D. (1997) 'Poverty and health', in D. Gordon and C. Pantazis (eds) *Breadline Britain in the 1990s*, Aldershot: Ashgate, pp 135-57.

Parker, H. (ed) (1998) *Low Cost but Acceptable: A minimum income standard for the UK: Families with young children*, Bristol: The Policy Press.

Patel, P., Mendall, M., Khulusi, S., Northfield, T.C. and Strachan, D.P. (1994) '*Helicobacter pylori* infection in childhood: risk factors and effect on growth', *BMJ*, vol 309, pp 1119-23.

Payne, S. (1997) 'Poverty and mental health', in D. Gordon and C. Pantazis (eds) *Breadline Britain in the 1990s*, Aldershot: Ashgate, pp 159-76.

Pearce, N.E., Davis, P.B., Smith, A.H. and Foster, F.H. (1983) 'Mortality and social class in New Zealand II: male mortality by major disease groupings', *New Zealand Medical Journal*, vol 96, pp 711-16.

Phillips, D.I., Barker, D.J., Hales, C.N., Hirst, S. and Osmond, C. (1994) 'Thinness at birth and insulin resistance in adult life', *Diabetologia*, vol 37, pp 150-4.

Pincus, T. and Callahan, L.F. (1994) 'Associations of low formal education level and poor health status: behavioural, in addition to demographic and medical, explanations?', *Journal of Clinical Epidemiology*, vol 47, pp 355-61.

Platt, S.D., Martin, C.J., Hunt, S. and Lewis, C.W. (1989) 'Damp housing, mold growth and symptomatic health state', *BMJ*, vol 298, pp 1673-8.

Pocock, S.J., Shaper, A.G., Cook, D.G., Phillips, A.N. and Walker, M. (1987) 'Social class differences in ischaemic heart disease in British men', *The Lancet*, vol 2, pp 197-201.

Power, C. and Matthews, S. (1997) 'Origins of health inequalities in a national population sample', *The Lancet*, vol 350, pp 1584-9.

Power, C., Manor, O. and Fox, A.J. (1991) *Health and class: The early years*, London: Chapman and Hall.

Power, C. Manor, O. and Matthews, S. (1999) 'The duration and timing of exposure: effects of socioeconomic environment on adult health', *American Journal of Public Health*, vol 89, no 7, pp 1059-65.

Power, C., Matthews, S. and Manor, O. (1996) 'Inequalities in self rated health in the 1958 birth cohort: life time social circumstances or social mobility?', *BMJ*, vol 313, pp 449-53.

Power, C., Matthews, S. and Manor, O. (1998) 'Inequalities in self-rated health: explanations from different stages of life', *The Lancet*, vol 351, pp 1009-14.

Power, C., Hertzman, C., Matthews, S. and Manor, O. (1997) 'Social differences in health: life-cycle effects between ages 23 and 33 in the 1958 British birth cohort', *American Journal of Public Health*, vol 87, pp 1499-503.

Power, S., Whitty, G. and Youdell, D. (1995) *No place to learn, homelessness and education*, London: Shelter,

Pryer, J.A., Brunner, E., Elliott, P., Nichols, R., Dimond, H. and Marmot, M. (1995) 'Who complied with COMA 1984 dietary fat recommendations among a nationally representative sample of British adults in 1986-7 and what do they eat?', *European Journal of Clinical Nutrition*, vol 49, pp 719-28.

Pullinger, J. (ed) (1998) *Social trends 28*, ONS, London: The Stationery Office.

Radical Statistics Health Group (1987) *Facing the figures*, London: Radical Statistics.

Raleigh, V.S. and Kiri, V.A. (1997) 'Life expectancy in England: variations and trends by gender, health authority, and level of deprivation', *Journal of Epidemiology and Community Health*, vol 51, pp 649-58.

Reading, R. (1997a) 'Social disadvantage and infection in childhood', *Sociology of Health and Illness*, vol 19, pp 395-414.

Reading, R. (1997b) 'Poverty and the health of children and adolescents', *Archives of Disease in Childhood*, vol 76, pp 463-7.

Reid, F. (1975) *The incomes of the blind: A review of the occupational and financial problems of blind people of all ages*, London: The Disability Alliance.

Roberts, I. and Power, C. (1996) 'Does the decline in child injury mortality vary by social class? A comparison of class specific mortality in 1981 and 1991', *BMJ*, vol 313, pp 784-6.

Robson, B., Bradford, M., Deas, I., Hall, E., Harrison, E., Parkinson, M., Evans, R., Garside, P., Harding, A. and Robinson, F. (1994) *Assessing the impact of urban policy*, London: HMSO.

Rutter, M. and Madge, N. (1976) *Cycles of disadvantage: A review of research*, London: Heinemann.

Salhi, M., Caselli, G., Duchène, J., Egidi, V., Santini, A., Thiltgès, E. and Wunsch, G. (1995) 'Assessing mortality differentials using life histories: a method and applications', in A. Lopez, G. Caselli and T. Valkonen (eds) *Adult mortality in developed countries: From description to explanation*, Oxford: Clarendon Press.

Salonen, J. (1982) 'Socioeconomic status and risk of cancer, cerebral stroke, and death due to coronary heart disease and any disease: a longitudinal study in eastern Finland', *Journal of Epidemiology and Community Health*, vol 36, pp 294-7.

Shaw, M. and Dorling, D. (1998) 'Mortality among street youth in the UK', *The Lancet*, vol 352, p 743.

Shelter (1998) *Growing up homeless*, London: Shelter.

Shouls, A., Congdon, P. and Curtis, S. (1998) 'Modelling inequality in reported long term illness: combining individual and area characteristics', *Journal of Epidemiology and Community Health*, vol 50, no 3, pp 366-76.

Simpson, S. and Dorling, D. (1994) 'Those missing millions: implications for social statistics of undercount in the 1991 census', *Journal of Social Policy*, vol 23, no 4, pp 543-67.

Smeeding, T.M. and Gottschalk, P. (1996) 'The international evidence on income distribution in modern economies: where do we stand?', in M. Kaser and Y. Mundlak (eds) *Contemporary economic development reviewed, Vol 2, Labour, food and poverty*, London: Oxford University Press.

Smith, J. and Harding, S. (1997) 'Mortality of women and men using alternative social classifications', in F. Drever and M. Whitehead (1997) *Health inequalities: Decennial supplement*, ONS, London: The Stationery Office.

Smyth, M. and Robus, N. (1989) *The financial circumstances of families with disabled children living in private households*, OPCS Surveys of Disability Report 5, London: HMSO.

Social Exclusion Unit (1998) *Truancy and school exclusion report*, London: Social Exclusion Unit.

Sooman, A., Macintyre, S. and Anderson, A. (1993) 'Scotland's health: a more difficult challenge for some?', *Health Bulletin*, vol 51, pp 276-84.

Stedman-Jones, G. (1984) *Outcast London*, London: Penguin.

Sterling, P. and Eyer, J. (1981) 'Biological basis of stress-related mortality', *Social Science and Medicine*, vol 15e, pp 3-42.

Susser, M.W., Watson, W. and Hooper, K. (1985) *Sociology in medicine*, Oxford: Oxford University Press.

Sutherland, H. (1999) *The impact of the 1999 Finance Bill on children*, London: Save the Children.

Syme, S.L. and Berkman, L.F. (1976) 'Social class, susceptibility and sickness', *American Journal of Epidemiology*, vol 104, pp 1-8.

Taylor, D.H. (1998) 'The natural life of policy indices: geographical problem areas in the US and UK', *Social Science and Medicine*, vol 6, pp 713-25.

The Sunday Times (1996) 'The rich list', 14 April.

The Times (1998) 'Rate of total exam failures up by half' [by John O'Leary], 27 August, p 1.

Thompson, E.J. (ed) (1975) *Social Trends No 6*, London: HMSO.

Thurlow, H.J. (1967) 'General susceptibility to illness: a selective review', *Canadian Medical Association Journal*, vol 97, pp 1397-404.

Totman, R. (1987) *Social causes of illness*, London: Souvenir Press.

Townsend, P. (1979) *Poverty in the United Kingdom*, London and Berkeley, CA: Allen Lane and Penguin, University of California Press.

Townsend, P. and Davidson, N. (1982) *Inequalities in health: The Black Report*, Harmondsworth: Penguin Books.

Townsend, P. and Davidson, N. (eds) (1988, 3rd edn, 1992) *Inequalities in health: The Black Report*; Whitehead, M. *(1988) The health divide*, London: Penguin Books.

Townsend, P., Corrigan, P. and Kowarzik, U. (1987) *Poverty and labour in London*, Interim Report of the Centenary Survey, London: Low Pay Unit.

Townsend, P., Phillimore, P. and Beattie, A. (1988) *Health and deprivation: Inequality and the North*, London: Croom Helm.

Tudor Hart, J. (1971) 'The inverse care law', *The Lancet*, vol 1, p 405.

Valkonen, T. (1987) 'Social inequality in the face of death', *European Population Conference 1987*, Helsinki: Central Statistical Office of Finland, pp 201-61.

Victor, C.R. (1997) 'The health of homeless people in Britain: a review', *European Journal of Public Health*, vol 7, pp 398-404.

Wadsworth, M. (1996) 'Family and education as determinants of health', in D. Blane, E. Brunner and R. Wilkinson (eds) *Health and social organization: Towards a health policy for the 21st century*, London: Routledge.

Wald, N., Kiryluk, S., Darby, S., Doll, R., Pike, M. and Peto, R. (eds) (1988) *UK smoking statistics*, Oxford: Oxford University Press.

Walker, E., Tobin, M. and McKennel, A. (1992) *Blind and partially sighted children in Britain: The RNIB Survey*, 2 Volumes, London: HMSO.

Wannamethee, S.G. and Shaper, A.G. (1997) 'Socioeconomic status within social class and mortality: a prospective study in middle-aged British men', *International Journal of Epidemiology*, vol 26, pp 532-41.

Wannamethee, S.G., Whincup, P.H., Shaper, G. and Walker, M. (1996) 'Influence of fathers' social class on cardiovascular disease in middle-aged men', *The Lancet*, vol 348, pp 1259-63.

Wiggins, R., Bartley, M., Gleave, S., Joshi, H., Lynch, K. and Mitchell, R. (1998) 'Limiting long-term illness: a question of where you live or who you are? A multilevel analysis of the 1971-1991 ONS Longitudinal Study', *Risk Decision and Policy*, vol 3, no 3, pp 181-98.

Wilkinson, R.G. (1989) 'Class mortality differentials, income and distribution and trends in poverty 1921-1981', *Journal of Social Policy*, vol 18, pp 307-35.

Wilkinson, R.G. (1990) 'Income distribution and mortality: a "natural" experiment', *Sociology of Health and Illness*, vol 12, pp 391-412.

Wilkinson, R.G. (1992) 'Income distribution and life expectancy', *BMJ*, vol 304, pp 65-8.

Winkleby, M.A., Jatulis, D.E., Frank, E. and Fortmann, S.P. (1992) 'Socioeconomic status and health: how education, income, and occupation contribute to risk factors for cardiovascular disease', *American Journal of Public Health*, vol 82, pp 816-20.

Whitehead, M. (1987) *The health divide: Inequalities in health in the 1980s*, London: Health Education Council.

WHO (World Health Organisation) (1998) *The World Health Report: Life in the 21st century: A vision for all*, Geneva: WHO.

WHO Europe (1999) *Health 21 – Health for all in the 21st century*, Copenhagen: WHO Regional Office for Europe.

Worrall, A., Rea, J. and Ben Shlomo, Y. (1997) 'Counting the cost of social disadvantage in primary care: retrospective analysis of patient data', *BMJ*, vol 314, pp 38-42.

Wrigley, N. (1998) 'How British retailers have shaped food choice', in A. Murcott (ed) *The nation's diet: The social science of food choice*, London: Longman.

Wunsch, G., Duchène, J., Thiltgès, E. and Salhi, M. (1996) 'Socioeconomic differences in mortality: a life course approach', *European Journal of Population*, vol 12, pp 167-85.

Zarb, G. and Maher, L. (1997) *The financial circumstance of disabled people in Northern Ireland*, PPRU Surveys of Disability Report 6, Belfast: Northern Ireland Statistics and Research Agency.

Appendix A: Premature mortality, poverty and avoidable deaths for each parliamentary constituency in Britain by Member of Parliament and their Party (1991-95)

The following table shows the SMRs (1991-95) for deaths under 65 for all of the 641 British constituencies. These are ranked by their SMR<65, and also divided into population groups of one million people aged under 65. The percentage of households in the constituency living in poverty in 1991 is also given. The column '% of avoidable deaths' refers to the percentage of deaths which would not have occurred had that constituency had the mortality rate of the best off health million. The Party and current (August 1999) Member of Parliament are given in the last two columns.

SMR rank	Name of constituency	SMR<65 1991-95	Poverty 1991	% avoidable deaths		Current MP as of August 1999
	'Worst health' million	178	37	62	Lab	14 of 15 MPs are Labour
	'Best health' million	68	13	0	Con	11 of 13 MPs are Conservative
	Britain	100	21	32	Lab	418 of 641 MPs are Labour
'Worst health' million						
1	Glasgow Shettleston	234	42	71	Lab	Mr David MARSHALL
2	Glasgow Springburn	217	41	69	Lab	Mr Michael MARTIN
3	Glasgow Maryhill	196	42	65	Lab	Mrs Maria FYFE
4	Glasgow Pollok	187	36	64	Lab	Mr Ian DAVIDSON
5	Glasgow Anniesland	181	34	63	Lab	The Rt Hon Donald DEWAR
6	Glasgow Baillieston	180	39	62	Lab	Mr Jimmy WRAY
7	Manchester Central	173	40	61	Lab	Mr Tony LLOYD
8	Glasgow Govan	172	31	61	Lab	Mr Mohammed SARWAR
9	Liverpool Riverside	172	39	61	Lab	Mrs Louise ELLMAN
10	Manchester Blackley	169	34	60	Lab	Mr Graham STRINGER
11	Greenock and Inverclyde	164	31	59	Lab	Dr Norman GODMAN
12	Salford	163	34	59	Lab	Ms Hazel BLEARS
13	Tyne Bridge	158	37	57	Lab	Mr David CLELLAND
14	Glasgow Kelvin	158	30	57	Lab	Mr George GALLOWAY
15	Southwark North and Bermondsey	156	38	56	Lib Dem	Mr Simon HUGHES

Population million number 2

16	Glasgow Rutherglen	156	30	56	Lab	Mr Tom McAVOY
17	Vauxhall	153	38	56	Lab	Ms Kate HOEY
18	Manchester Gorton	153	32	56	Lab	The Rt Hon Gerald KAUFMAN
19	Glasgow Cathcart	151	31	55	Lab	Mr John MAXTON
20	Hamilton North and Bellshill	150	30	55	Lab	Dr John REID
21	Holborn and St Pancras	150	36	55	Lab	Mr Frank DOBSON
22	Birmingham Ladywood	148	38	54	Lab	Ms Clare SHORT
23	Airdrie and Shotts	148	34	54	Lab	Mrs Helen LIDDELL
24	Poplar and Canning Town	146	37	54	Lab	Mr Jim FITZPATRICK
25	Motherwell and Wishaw	146	34	53	Lab	Mr Frank ROY
26	Middlesbrough	145	29	53	Lab	Mr Stuart BELL
27	Birkenhead	144	28	53	Lab	Mr Frank FIELD
28	Birmingham Sparkbrook and Small Heath	143	32	53	Lab	Mr Roger GODSIFF
29	Coatbridge and Chryston	143	32	53	Lab	Mr Tom CLARKE

Population million number 3

30	Paisley North	143	31	53	Lab	Ms Irene ADAMS
31	Bootle	142	33	52	Lab	Mr Joe BENTON
32	Leeds Central	142	35	52	Lab	Mr Derek FATCHETT
33	Edinburgh North and Leith	142	25	52	Lab	Mr Malcolm CHISHOLM
34	Hamilton South	142	30	52	Lab	Mr George ROBERTSON
35	Bethnal Green and Bow	141	38	52	Lab	Ms Oona KING
36	Paisley South	141	31	52	Lab	Mr Gordon McMASTER
37	Birmingham Erdington	141	29	52	Lab	Mr Robin CORBETT
38	Liverpool West Derby	141	33	52	Lab	Mr Robert WAREING
39	Dundee West	139	33	51	Lab	Mr Ernie ROSS
40	Camberwell and Peckham	139	39	51	Lab	Ms Harriet HARMAN
41	Hackney South and Shoreditch	138	39	51	Lab	Mr Brian SEDGEMORE
42	Liverpool Walton	138	33	51	Lab	Mr Peter KILFOYLE

Population million number 4

43	Edinburgh Central	137	24	50	Lab	Mr Alistair DARLING
44	Stoke Central	137	26	50	Lab	Mr Mark FISHER
45	Preston	136	26	50	Lab	Mrs Audrey WISE
46	Dundee East	136	31	50	Lab	Mr John McALLION
47	Easington	136	29	50	Lab	Mr John CUMMINGS
48	Cunninghame South	135	32	50	Lab	Mr Brian DONOHOE
49	Nottingham East	134	30	49	Lab	Mr John HEPPELL
50	Blackpool South	134	23	49	Lab	Mr Gordon MARSDEN
51	Hackney North and Stoke Newington	133	36	49	Lab	Ms Diane ABBOTT
52	Hammersmith and Fulham	133	28	49	Lab	Mr Iain COLEMAN
53	Bradford West	133	27	49	Lab	Mr Marsha SINGH
54	Bolton South East	132	26	49	Lab	Dr Brian IDDON
55	Wythenshawe and Sale East	131	31	48	Lab	Mr Paul GOGGINS

Population million number 5

56	Newcastle East and Wallsend	131	32	48	Lab	Mr Nick BROWN
57	Rochdale	130	27	48	Lab	Ms Lorna FITZSIMMONS
58	Regents Park and Kensington North	130	33	48	Lab	Ms Karen BUCK
59	Blackburn	130	25	48	Lab	Mr Jack STRAW
60	Stockton North	130	26	48	Lab	Mr Frank COOK
61	Dumbarton	129	26	48	Lab	Mr John McFALL
62	Argyll and Bute	129	26	47	Lib Dem	Mrs Ray MICHIE

63	Houghton and Washington East	129	28	47	Lab	Mr Fraser KEMP
64	Islington South and Finsbury	128	37	47	Lab	Mr Chris SMITH
65	West Ham	128	32	47	Lab	Mr Tony BANKS
66	Jarrow	128	29	47	Lab	Mr Stephen HEPBURN
67	Aberdeen Central	128	29	47	Lab	Mr Frank DORAN
68	Cunninghame North	128	25	47	Lab	Mr Brian WILSON

Population million number 6

69	Wallasey	127	23	47	Lab	Ms Angela EAGLE
70	Ashton under Lyne	127	25	47	Lab	The Rt Hon Robert SHELDON
71	Western Isles	127	23	47	Lab	Mr Calum MacDONALD
72	Clydebank and Milngavie	127	28	47	Lab	Mr Tony WORTHINGTON
73	South Shields	127	31	47	Lab	Dr David CLARK
74	Islington North	127	35	47	Lab	Mr Jeremy CORBYN
75	Bradford North	127	26	46	Lab	Mr Terry ROONEY
76	Edinburgh East and Musselburgh	126	25	46	Lab	Dr Gavin STRANG
77	Rhondda	126	25	46	Lab	Mr Allan ROGERS
78	Hartlepool	126	27	46	Lab	Mr Peter MANDELSON
79	Acton and Shepherds Bush	126	28	46	Lab	Mr Clive SOLEY
80	Burnley	126	23	46	Lab	Mr Peter PIKE
81	Wolverhampton South East	126	29	46	Lab	Mr Dennis TURNER
82	Hull East	125	30	46	Lab	The Rt Hon John PRESCOTT

Population million number 7

83	Eccles	125	25	46	Lab	Mr Ian STEWART
84	Sunderland North	125	30	46	Lab	Mr Bill ETHERINGTON
85	Sheffield Central	125	34	46	Lab	Mr Richard CABORN
86	Sheffield Brightside	125	34	46	Lab	Mr David BLUNKETT
87	Falkirk West	124	29	46	Lab	Mr Dennis CANAVAN
88	Birmingham Hodge Hill	124	30	45	Lab	Mr Terry DAVIS
89	Great Grimsby	124	24	45	Lab	Mr Austin MITCHELL
90	Walsall North	124	28	45	Lab	Mr David WINNICK
91	Manchester Withington	123	26	45	Lab	Mr Keith BRADLEY
92	Knowsley South	123	29	45	Lab	Mr Eddie O'HARA
93	Streatham	123	29	45	Lab	Mr Keith HILL
94	Liverpool Garston	123	27	45	Lab	Ms Maria EAGLE
95	Tottenham	123	33	45	Lab	Mr Bernie GRANT

Population million number 8

96	Leeds East	123	29	45	Lab	Mr George MUDIE
97	Nottingham North	123	30	45	Lab	Mr Graham ALLEN
98	Liverpool Wavertree	122	27	45	Lab	Mrs Jane KENNEDY
99	Merthyr Tydfil and Rhymney	122	31	45	Lab	Mr Ted ROWLANDS
100	West Bromwich West	122	29	45	Speaker	Ms Betty BOOTHROYD
101	Warley	122	27	44	Lab	Mr John SPELLAR
102	Deptford	122	32	44	Lab	Mrs Joan RUDDOCK
103	Stoke North	122	23	44	Lab	Mrs Joan WALLEY
104	Kilmarnock and Loudoun	121	28	44	Lab	Mr Desmond BROWN
105	Caithness Sutherland and Easter Ross	121	27	44	Lib Dem	Mr Robert MacLENNAN
106	Halifax	121	23	44	Lab	Mrs Alice MAHON
107	Oldham West and Royton	121	25	44	Lab	Mr Michael MEACHER
108	Leicester West	121	28	44	Lab	Ms Patricia HEWITT
109	Cynon Valley	120	25	44	Lab	Mrs Ann CLWYD

Population million number 9

110	Midlothian	120	27	44	Lab	Mr Eric CLARKE
111	Dunfermline West	120	22	44	Lab	Ms Rachel SQUIRE
112	West Bromwich East	120	26	44	Lab	Mr Peter SNAPE
113	Newcastle Central	120	28	44	Lab	Mr Jim COUSINS
114	Blackpool North and Fleetwood	120	20	43	Lab	Mrs Joan HUMBLE
115	Sunderland South	120	30	43	Lab	Mr Chris MULLIN
116	Stirling	120	22	43	Lab	Mrs Anne McGUIRE
117	Perth	120	22	43	SNP	Ms Roseanna CUNNINGHAM
118	Greenwich and Woolwich	120	32	43	Lab	Mr Nick RAYNSFORD
119	Walsall South	120	25	43	Lab	Mr Bruce GEORGE
120	Cardiff South and Penarth	119	25	43	Lab	Mr Alun MICHAEL
121	Galloway and Upper Nithsdale	119	25	43	SNP	Mr Alasdair MORGAN
122	Bolton North East	119	23	43	Lab	Mr David CRAUSBY
123	Hull West and Hessle	119	29	43	Lab	Alan JOHNSON
124	Redcar	119	25	43	Lab	Dr Mo MOWLAM

Population million number 10

125	Cumbernauld and Kilsyth	119	25	43	Lab	Ms Rosemary MCKENNA
126	Barnsley Central	119	27	43	Lab	Mr Eric ILLSLEY
127	Darlington	118	23	43	Lab	Mr Alan MILBURN
128	Battersea	118	27	43	Lab	Mr Martin LINTON
129	Oldham East and Saddleworth	118	21	43	Lab	Mr Phil WOOLAS
130	West Renfrewshire	118	22	43	Lab	Mr Tommy GRAHAM
131	Carrick Cumnock and Doon Valley	118	28	43	Lab	Mr George FOULKES
132	St Helens South	118	24	43	Lab	Mr Gerry BERMINGHAM
133	Dulwich and West Norwood	118	27	43	Lab	Ms Tessa JOWELL
134	Central Fife	118	27	43	Lab	Mr Henry McLEISH
135	Heywood and Middleton	118	23	42	Lab	Mr Jim DOBBIN
136	Barking	118	29	42	Lab	Ms Margaret HODGE
137	Kirkcaldy	118	26	42	Lab	Dr Lewis MOONIE

Population million number 11

138	Coventry North East	118	25	42	Lab	Mr Bob AINSWORTH
139	East Ham	117	28	42	Lab	Mr Stephen TIMMS
140	Knowsley North and Sefton East	117	26	42	Lab	Mr George HOWARTH
141	North Tyneside	117	30	42	Lab	Mr Stephen BYERS
142	Bradford South	117	23	42	Lab	Mr Gerry SUTCLIFFE
143	North West Durham	117	24	42	Lab	Ms Hilary ARMSTRONG
144	Ayr	117	23	42	Lab	Ms Sandra OSBOURNE
145	Doncaster North	117	26	42	Lab	Mr Kevin HUGHES
146	Brent East	117	29	42	Lab	Mr Ken LIVINGSTONE
147	Stockport	117	21	42	Lab	Ms Ann COFFEY
148	Linlithgow	117	28	42	Lab	Mr Tam DALYELL
149	Swansea East	117	25	42	Lab	Mr Donald ANDERSON
150	Brent South	117	29	42	Lab	Mr Paul BOATENG
151	Carlisle	116	23	42	Lab	Mr Eric MARTLEW

Population million number 12

152	Wolverhampton North East	116	27	42	Lab	Mr Ken PURCHASE
153	Brighton Kemptown	116	22	42	Lab	Dr Desmond TURNER
154	Lincoln	116	23	41	Lab	Ms Gillian MERRON
155	Pontefract and Castleford	116	27	41	Lab	Ms Yvette COOPER

156	Sedgefield	116	25	41	Lab	The Rt Hon Tony BLAIR
157	Nottingham South	115	27	41	Lab	Mr Alan SIMPSON
158	Leicester East	115	25	41	Lab	Mr Keith VAZ
159	Aberavon	115	24	41	Lab	The Rt Hon John MORRIS
160	Warrington North	115	20	41	Lab	Ms Helen JONES
161	Cardiff West	115	24	41	Lab	Mr Rhodri MORGAN
162	Halton	115	23	41	Lab	Mr John TWIGG
163	Dunfermline East	114	28	41	Lab	The Rt Hon Gordon BROWN
164	Hyndburn	114	20	41	Lab	Mr Greg POPE
165	Blaenau Gwent	114	27	41	Lab	Mr Llew SMITH

Population million number 13

166	Livingston	114	25	41	Lab	The Rt Hon Robin COOK
167	Neath	114	22	41	Lab	Mr Peter HAIN
168	Ross Skye and Inverness West	114	24	41	Lib Dem	Mr Charles KENNEDY
169	Clydesdale	114	26	41	Lab	Mr Jimmy HOOD
170	Ochil	114	25	41	Lab	Mr Martin O'NEILL
171	Ogmore	113	23	40	Lab	Sir Ray POWELL
172	Stalybridge and Hyde	113	23	40	Lab	Mr Tom PENDRY
173	Huddersfield	113	26	40	Lab	Mr Barry SHEERMAN
174	Bishop Auckland	113	24	40	Lab	The Rt Hon Derek FOSTER
175	Tooting	113	24	40	Lab	Mr Tom COX
176	East Kilbride	113	22	40	Lab	Mr Adam INGRAM
177	Plymouth Sutton	113	25	40	Lab	Mrs Linda GILROY
178	Southall	113	22	40	Lab	Mr Piara KHABRA
179	Worsley	113	23	40	Lab	Mr Terry LEWIS

Population million number 14

180	Luton South	113	20	40	Lab	Ms Margaret MORAN
181	Aberdeen North	112	25	40	Lab	Mr Malcolm SAVIDGE
182	Torfaen	112	25	40	Lab	Mr Paul MURPHY
183	Wansbeck	112	25	40	Lab	Mr Dennis MURPHY
184	Lewisham East	112	27	40	Lab	Mrs Bridget PRENTICE
185	Leeds West	112	28	40	Lab	Mr John BATTLE
186	Gateshead East and Washington West	112	29	40	Lab	Ms Joyce QUIN
187	Scunthorpe	112	22	39	Lab	Mr Elliot MORLEY
188	Middlesbrough South and East Cleveland	112	22	39	Lab	Dr Ashok KUMAR
189	Coventry South	111	22	39	Lab	Mr Jim CUNNINGHAM
190	Corby	111	21	39	Lab	Mr Philip HOPE
191	Rotherham	111	28	39	Lab	Dr Denis MacSHANE
192	Copeland	111	22	39	Lab	The Rt Hon Jack CUNNINGHAM
193	Birmingham Selly Oak	111	23	39	Lab	Dr Lynne JONES

Population million number 15

194	Leigh	111	23	39	Lab	Mr Lawrie CUNLIFFE
195	Stoke South	111	22	39	Lab	Mr George STEVENSON
196	Derby South	111	23	39	Lab	The Rt Hon Margaret BECKETT
197	Barrow and Furness	111	19	39	Lab	Mr John HUTTON
198	Portsmouth South	111	25	39	Lib Dem	Mr Mike HANCOCK
199	Barnsley East and Mexborough	110	26	39	Lab	Mr Jeff ENNIS
200	Vale of Clwyd	110	20	39	Lab	Mr Chris RUANE
201	Southampton Test	110	23	38	Lab	Dr Alan WHITEHEAD
202	Walthamstow	110	26	38	Lab	Mr Neil GERRARD
203	Leicester South	109	27	38	Lab	Mr James MARSHALL

204	Newport East	109	21	38	Lab	Mr Alan HOWARTH
205	Denton and Reddish	109	22	38	Lab	Mr Andrew BENNETT

Population million number 16

206	Slough	109	20	38	Lab	Ms Fiona MacTAGGART
207	Rossendale and Darwen	109	18	38	Lab	Mrs Janet ANDERSON
208	Birmingham Edgbaston	109	25	38	Lab	Ms Gisela STUART
209	Birmingham Yardley	108	24	37	Lab	Ms Estelle MORRIS
210	Chesterfield	108	23	37	Lab	The Rt Hon Tony BENN
211	Southampton Itchen	108	23	37	Lab	Mr John DENHAM
212	Birmingham Northfield	108	26	37	Lab	Mr Richard BURDEN
213	Makerfield	108	21	37	Lab	Mr Ian McCARTNEY
214	Doncaster Central	108	25	37	Lab	Ms Rosalie WINTERTON
215	North Thanet	108	20	37	Con	Mr Roger GALE
216	Stretford and Urmston	108	22	37	Lab	Ms Beverley HUGHES
217	Birmingham Perry Barr	108	22	37	Lab	Mr Jeff ROOKER
218	Pendle	107	20	37	Lab	Mr Gordon PRENTICE
219	Edinburgh South	107	22	37	Lab	Mr Nigel GRIFFITHS

Population million number 17

220	Dumfries	107	23	37	Lab	Mr Russell BROWN
221	Dagenham	107	26	37	Lab	Ms Judith CHURCH
222	Carmarthen East and Dinefwr	107	18	37	Lab	Dr Alan W. WILLIAMS
223	Plymouth Devonport	107	25	37	Lab	Mr David JAMIESON
224	Wentworth	107	25	37	Lab	Mr John HEALY
225	Ynys Mon	107	19	37	Plaid Cymru	Mr Ieuan Wyn JONES
226	Llanelli	107	22	37	Lab	The Rt Hon Denzil DAVIES
227	Swansea West	107	24	36	Lab	The Rt Hon Alan J. WILLIAMS
228	St Helens North	106	22	36	Lab	Mr John EVANS
229	Workington	106	21	36	Lab	Mr Dale CAMPBELL-SAVOURS
230	Putney	106	24	36	Lab	Mr Anthony COLMAN
231	Bolsover	106	22	36	Lab	Mr Dennis SKINNER
232	Hemsworth	106	24	36	Lab	Mr Jon TRICKETT
233	Dewsbury	105	23	36	Lab	Mrs Ann TAYLOR

Population million number 18

234	Moray	105	22	36	SNP	Ms Margaret EWING
235	Hampstead and Highgate	105	28	36	Lab	Ms Glenda JACKSON
236	Brighton Pavilion	105	22	36	Lab	Mr David LEPPER
237	Falkirk East	105	26	36	Lab	Mr Michael CONNARTY
238	Coventry North West	105	19	36	Lab	Mr Geoffrey ROBINSON
239	Morecambe and Lunesdale	105	19	35	Lab	Ms Geraldine SMITH
240	Wrexham	105	23	35	Lab	Dr John MAREK
241	Thurrock	105	21	35	Lab	Mr Andrew MacKINLAY
242	Hull North	105	29	35	Lab	Mr Kevin McNAMARA
243	Southport	105	17	35	Lib Dem	Mr Ronnie FEARN
244	Caerphilly	105	23	35	Lab	Mr Ron DAVIES
245	Newcastle under Lyme	105	21	35	Lab	Mrs Llin GOLDING
246	Newport West	105	23	35	Lab	Mr Paul FLYNN
247	Angus	105	22	35	SNP	Mr Andrew WELSH
248	Delyn	104	18	35	Lab	Mr David HANSON

Population million number 19

249	Tynemouth	104	21	35	Lab	Mr Alan CAMPBELL
250	Wigan	104	23	35	Lab	Mr Roger STOTT
251	Sheffield Heeley	104	29	35	Lab	Mr Bill MICHIE

252	Bury South	104	19	35	Lab	Mr Ivan LEWIS
253	Boston and Skegness	104	20	35	Con	Sir Richard BODY
254	Birmingham Hall Green	104	22	35	Lab	Mr Stephen McCABE
255	Brigg and Goole	104	18	35	Lab	Mr Ian CAWSEY
256	Rochford and Southend East	104	20	35	Con	Sir Teddy TAYLOR
257	Inverness East Nairn and Lochaber	104	21	35	Lab	Mr David STEWART
258	Derby North	104	20	35	Lab	Mr Bob LAXTON
259	Dudley North	104	24	35	Lab	The Rt Hon Dr John GILBERT
260	Lewisham West	104	26	35	Lab	Mr Jim DOWD
261	Bristol South	104	24	35	Lab	Ms Dawn PRIMAROLO

Population million number 20

262	Batley and Spen	103	21	35	Lab	Mr Mike WOOD
263	Hayes and Harlington	103	19	34	Lab	Mr John McDONNELL
264	Ellesmere Port and Neston	103	19	34	Lab	Mr Andrew MILLER
265	Leyton and Wanstead	103	25	34	Lab	Mr Harry COHEN
266	Banff and Buchan	103	25	34	SNP	Mr Alex SALMOND
267	Louth and Horncastle	103	16	34	Con	Sir Peter TAPSELL
268	Wolverhampton South West	103	21	34	Lab	Mrs Jenny JONES
269	Preseli Pembrokeshire	103	19	34	Lab	Ms Jackie LAWRENCE
270	Croydon North	103	21	34	Lab	Mr Malcolm WICKS
271	Newcastle North	102	25	34	Lab	Mr Doug HENDERSON
272	Stockton South	102	18	34	Lab	Ms Daria TAYLOR
273	Blyth Valley	102	23	34	Lab	Mr Ronnie CAMPBELL
274	Mansfield	102	22	34	Lab	Mr Alan MEALE
275	Barnsley West and Penistone	102	23	34	Lab	Mr Michael CLAPHAM

Population million number 21

276	Hove	102	21	34	Lab	Mr Ivor CAPLIN
277	Hastings and Rye	102	21	33	Lab	Mr Michael FOSTER
278	Sheffield Attercliffe	102	24	33	Lab	Mr Clive BETTS
279	Islwyn	102	22	33	Lab	Mr Don TOUHIG
280	Clwyd South	102	22	33	Lab	Mr Martyn JONES
281	Bristol East	102	21	33	Lab	Ms Jean CORSTON
282	Feltham and Heston	102	21	33	Lab	Mr Alan KEEN
283	Roxburgh and Berwickshire	102	25	33	Lib Dem	Mr Archy KIRKWOOD
284	Bassetlaw	102	21	33	Lab	Mr Joe ASHTON
285	Cannock Chase	102	19	33	Lab	Dr Tony WRIGHT
286	Normanton	101	20	33	Lab	Mr William O'BRIEN
287	Bournemouth East	101	18	33	Con	David ATKINSON
288	City of York	101	23	33	Lab	Mr Hugh BAYLEY
289	Blaydon	101	24	33	Lab	Mr John McWILLIAM

Population million number 22

290	Newark	101	19	33	Lab	Mrs Fiona JONES
291	Dover	101	20	33	Lab	Mr Gwyn PROSSER
292	Oxford East	101	24	33	Lab	Mr Andrew SMITH
293	Cleethorpes	101	18	33	Lab	Ms Shona McISAAC
294	Bognor Regis and Littlehampton	101	17	33	Con	Mr Nicolas GIBB
295	Amber Valley	101	18	33	Lab	Ms Judy MALLABER
296	Erith and Thamesmead	100	25	33	Lab	Mr John AUSTIN-WALKER
297	Harwich	100	18	32	Lab	Mr Ivan HENDERSON
298	Brentford and Isleworth	100	21	32	Lab	Ms Ann KEEN
299	Great Yarmouth	100	21	32	Lab	Mr Tony WRIGHT
300	North Durham	100	24	32	Lab	Mr Giles RADICE
301	Wakefield	100	22	32	Lab	Mr David HINCHLIFFE

| 302 | East Lothian | 100 | 25 | 32 | Lab | Mr John HOME ROBERTSON |
| 303 | Caernarfon | 100 | 19 | 32 | Plaid Cymru | Mr Dafydd WIGLEY |

Population million number 23

304	Rother Valley	100	21	32	Lab	Mr Kevin BARRON
305	Alyn and Deeside	100	17	32	Lab	Mr Barry JONES
306	Gloucester	99	18	32	Lab	Ms Tess KINGHAM
307	Pontypridd	99	19	32	Lab	Dr Kim HOWELLS
308	Warrington South	99	16	32	Lab	Mrs Helen SOUTHWORTH
309	North East Cambridgeshire	99	17	32	Con	Mr Malcolm MOSS
310	Milton Keynes South West	99	20	31	Lab	Dr Phyllis STARKEY
311	Calder Valley	99	19	31	Lab	Ms Christine McCAFFERTY
312	Falmouth and Camborne	99	19	31	Lab	Ms Candy ATHERTON
313	Strathkelvin and Bearsden	99	16	31	Lab	Mr Sam GALBRAITH
314	Ashfield	98	21	31	Lab	Mr Geoff HOON
315	Mitcham and Morden	98	21	31	Lab	Ms Siobhan McDONAGH
316	Conwy	98	21	31	Lab	Mrs Betty WILLIAMS

Population million number 24

317	Bridgend	98	18	31	Lab	Mr Win GRIFFITHS
318	Orkney and Shetland	98	22	31	Lib Dem	Mr James WALLACE
319	Medway	98	18	31	Lab	Mr Robert MARSHALL-ANDREWS
320	City of Chester	98	20	31	Lab	Ms Christine RUSSELL
321	Don Valley	98	21	31	Lab	Ms Caroline FLINT
322	Ribble Valley	98	12	31	Con	Mr Nigel EVANS
323	Merionnydd nant Conwy	98	18	31	Plaid Cymru	Mr Elfyn LLWYD
324	Weaver Vale	98	21	31	Lab	Mr Mike HALL
325	Havant	98	19	31	Con	Mr David WILLETTS
326	Halesowen and Rowley Regis	98	21	31	Lab	Mrs Sylvia HEAL
327	Bristol North West	98	21	31	Lab	Dr Doug NAYSMITH
328	Portsmouth North	98	20	31	Lab	Mr Syd RAPSON
329	Burton	97	19	31	Lab	Mrs Janet DEAN
330	Aberdeen South	97	20	31	Lab	Miss Anne BEGG
331	Crosby	97	16	30	Lab	Ms Claire CURTIS-TANSLEY

Population million number 25

332	North Tayside	97	22	30	SNP	Mr John SWINNEY
333	Waveney	97	19	30	Lab	Mr Bob BLIZZARD
334	Northampton North	97	21	30	Lab	Ms Sally KEEBLE
335	Hornsey and Wood Green	97	25	30	Lab	Mrs Barbara ROCHE
336	Worcester	97	19	30	Lab	Mr Michael FOSTER
337	Bury North	97	18	30	Lab	Mr David CHAYTOR
338	Edinburgh West	97	18	30	Lib Dem	Mr Donald GORRIE
339	Morley and Rothwell	96	22	30	Lab	Mr John GUNNELL
340	Ceredigion	96	17	30	Plaid Cymru	Mr Cynog DAFIS
341	Brecon and Radnorshire	96	18	30	Lib Dem	Mr Richard LIVSEY
342	Staffordshire Moorlands	96	16	30	Lab	Ms Charlotte ATKINS
343	Clwyd West	96	17	30	Lab	Mr Gareth THOMAS
344	Peterborough	96	22	30	Lab	Mrs Helen BRINTON
345	Northampton South	96	17	30	Lab	Mr Tony CLARKE

Population million number 26

346	Torbay	96	19	30	Lib Dem	Mr Adrian SANDERS
347	South Thanet	96	20	30	Lab	Dr Stephen LADYMAN
348	South Holland and the Deepings	96	16	30	Con	Mr John HAYES

349	The Wrekin	96	19	30	Lab	Mr Peter BRADLEY
350	Edinburgh Pentlands	96	20	29	Lab	Dr Lynda CLARK
351	Berwick upon Tweed	96	23	29	Lib Dem	The Rt Hon Alan BEITH
352	Edmonton	96	22	29	Lab	Mr Andrew LOVE
353	Telford	96	21	29	Lab	Mr Bruce GROCOTT
354	Exeter	96	20	29	Lab	Mr Ben BRADSHAW
355	Fylde	96	16	29	Con	Mr Michael JACK
356	Stone	96	14	29	Con	Mr Bill CASH
357	Scarborough and Whitby	95	21	29	Lab	Mr Lawrie QUINN
358	Carmarthen West and South Pembrokeshire	95	19	29	Lab	Mr Nick AINGER
359	Ipswich	95	22	29	Lab	Mr Jamie CANN

Population million number 27

360	Sittingbourne and Sheppey	95	18	29	Lab	Mr Derek WYATT
361	Crewe and Nantwich	95	19	29	Lab	Mrs Gwyneth DUNWOODY
362	Cities of London and Westminster	95	31	29	Con	The Rt Hon Peter BROOKE
363	Keighley	95	18	29	Lab	Ms Ann CRYER
364	Bournemouth West	95	20	29	Con	Mr John BUTTERFILL
365	West Lancashire	95	20	29	Lab	Mr Colin PICKTHALL
366	Dudley South	95	20	29	Lab	Mr Ian PEARSON
367	Erewash	95	18	29	Lab	Ms Elizabeth BLACKMAN
368	East Yorkshire	95	18	29	Con	Mr John TOWNEND
369	Kensington and Chelsea	95	25	29	Con	Mr Allan CLARK
370	Luton North	95	18	29	Lab	Mr Kelvin HOPKINS
371	Bedford	95	19	28	Lab	Mr Patrick HALL
372	Lancaster and Wyre	95	15	28	Lab	Mr Thomas DAWSON

Population million number 28

373	Shipley	95	17	28	Lab	Mr Christopher LESLIE
374	Poole	95	17	28	Con	Mr Robert SYMS
375	Ilford South	94	17	28	Lab	Mr Mike GAPES
376	North East Fife	94	19	28	Lib Dem	Mr Menzies CAMPBELL
377	Warwick and Leamington	94	18	28	Lab	Mr James PLASKITT
378	Colne Valley	94	17	28	Lab	Ms Kali MOUNTFORD
379	Nuneaton	94	18	28	Lab	Mr Bill OLNER
380	Sherwood	94	17	28	Lab	Mr Paddy TIPPING
381	City of Durham	94	23	28	Lab	Mr Gerry STEINBERG
382	Bristol West	94	18	28	Lab	Ms Valerie DAVEY
383	Tamworth	93	18	27	Lab	Mr Brian JENKINS
384	St Ives	93	19	27	Lib Dem	Mr Andrew GEORGE
385	South Ribble	93	14	27	Lab	Mr David BORROW

Population million number 29

386	Montgomeryshire	93	18	27	Lib Dem	Mr Lembit OPIK
387	Cardiff Central	93	21	27	Lab	Mr Jon Owen JONES
388	Norwich South	93	25	27	Lab	Mr Charles CLARKE
389	Worthing West	93	16	27	Con	Mr Peter BOTTOMLEY
390	Gainsborough	93	17	27	Con	Mr Edward LEIGH
391	Eddisbury	93	16	27	Con	The Rt Hon Alistair GOODLAD
392	Gordon	93	17	27	Lib Dem	Mr Malcolm BRUCE
393	Cheltenham	92	19	27	Lib Dem	Mr Nigel JONES
394	South Dorset	92	18	27	Con	Mr Ian BRUCE
395	Chatham and Aylesford	92	15	27	Lab	Mr Jonathan SHAW
396	Forest of Dean	92	16	26	Lab	Mrs Diana ORGAN
397	High Peak	92	17	26	Lab	Mr Tom LEVITT
398	Folkestone and Hythe	92	19	26	Con	The Rt Hon Michael HOWARD

| 399 | Truro and St Austell | 92 | 17 | 26 | Lib Dem | Mr Matthew TAYLOR |

Population million number 30

400	Cardiff North	92	15	26	Lab	Ms Julie MORGAN
401	Gower	92	17	26	Lab	Mr Martin CATON
402	Swindon South	92	18	26	Lab	Ms Julia DROWN
403	Dartford	92	16	26	Lab	Dr Howard STOATE
404	Grantham and Stamford	92	18	26	Con	Mr Quentin DAVIES
405	Weston super Mare	92	17	26	Lib Dem	Mr Brian COTTER
406	Vale of Glamorgan	92	17	26	Lab	Mr John SMITH
407	Harrogate and Knaresborough	92	16	26	Lib Dem	Mr Phil WILLIS
408	Wyre Forest	91	17	26	Lab	Mr David LOCK
409	Bolton West	91	17	26	Lab	Ms Ruth KELLY
410	North West Norfolk	91	18	26	Lab	Mr George TURNER
411	Harlow	91	23	26	Lab	Mr Bill RAMMELL
412	North Warwickshire	91	18	26	Lab	Mr Mike O'BRIEN

Population million number 31

413	Eastbourne	91	19	26	Con	Mr Nigel WATERSON
414	Isle of Wight	91	18	25	Lib Dem	Dr Peter BRAND
415	Leeds North East	91	20	25	Lab	Mr Fabian HAMILTON
416	Eltham	91	23	25	Lab	Mr Clive EFFORD
417	Hazel Grove	91	16	25	Lib Dem	Mr Andrew STUNELL
418	South Derbyshire	91	16	25	Lab	Mr Mark TODD
419	Croydon Central	91	19	25	Lab	Cllr Geraint DAVIES
420	Penrith and the Border	91	15	25	Con	The Rt Hon David MacLEAN
421	Hornchurch	91	15	25	Lab	Mr John CRYER
422	North Shropshire	91	18	25	Con	Mr Owen PATERSON
423	Carshalton and Wallington	90	18	25	Lib Dem	Mr Tom BRAKE
424	North East Derbyshire	90	20	25	Lab	Mr Harry BARNES
425	Wirral West	90	16	25	Lab	Mr Stephen HESFORD

Population million number 32

426	Basildon	90	20	25	Lab	Ms Angela SMITH
427	Tweeddale Ettrick and Lauderdale	90	21	25	Lib Dem	Mr Michael MOORE
428	Wells	90	15	25	Con	The Rt Hon David HEATHCOAT-AMORY
429	Ealing North	90	20	25	Lab	Mr Stephen POUND
430	Sheffield Hillsborough	90	20	24	Lab	Mrs Helen JACKSON
431	Torridge and West Devon	90	16	24	Lib Dem	Mr John BURNETT
432	Crawley	89	20	24	Lab	Mrs Laura MOFFATT
433	Gosport	89	17	24	Con	Mr Peter VIGGERS
434	Ilford North	89	17	24	Lab	Ms Linda PERHAM
435	Reading West	89	17	24	Lab	Mr Martin SALTER
436	Gedling	89	16	24	Lab	Mr Vernon COAKER
437	Rugby and Kenilworth	89	16	24	Lab	Mr Andrew KING
438	Upminster	89	17	24	Lab	Mr Keith DARVILL

Population million number 33

439	Tatton	89	14	23	Ind	Mr Martin BELL
440	Colchester	88	19	23	Lib Dem	Mr Bob RUSSELL
441	Taunton	88	17	23	Lib Dem	Mrs Jackie BALLARD
442	Chorley	88	16	23	Lab	Ms Lindsey HOYLE
443	Gravesham	88	19	23	Lab	Mr Chris POND
444	Altrincham and Sale West	88	15	23	Con	Mr Graham BRADY

445	Teignbridge	88	15	23	Con	Mr Patrick NICHOLLS
446	Aldridge-Brownhills	88	18	23	Con	Mr Richard SHEPHERD
447	North Devon	88	17	23	Lib Dem	Mr Nick HARVEY
448	Meriden	88	20	23	Con	Ms Caroline SPELMAN
449	North Cornwall	87	17	23	Lib Dem	Mr Paul TYLER
450	Enfield North	87	19	22	Lab	Ms Joan RYAN
451	Shrewsbury and Atcham	87	17	22	Lab	Mr Paul MARSDEN

Population million number 34

452	Swindon North	87	18	22	Lab	Mr Michael WILLS
453	South West Norfolk	87	17	22	Con	The Rt Hon Mrs Gillian SHEPHARD
454	Salisbury	87	18	22	Con	Mr Robert KEY
455	Reigate	87	14	22	Con	Mr Crispin BLUNT
456	West Dorset	87	16	22	Con	Dr Oliver LETWIN
457	North West Leicestershire	87	17	22	Lab	Mr David TAYLOR
458	North East Bedfordshire	87	14	22	Con	The Rt Hon Sir Nicholas LYELL
459	Worthing East and Shoreham	87	16	22	Con	Mr Timothy LOUGHTON
460	Elmet	87	17	22	Lab	Mr Colin BURGON
461	Stafford	87	17	22	Lab	Mr David KIDNEY
462	Eastwood	86	15	22	Lab	Mr Jim MURPHY
463	Wirral South	86	15	22	Lab	Mr Ben CHAPMAN
464	Hereford	86	19	21	Lib Dem	Mr Paul KEETCH
465	Brent North	86	16	21	Lab	Mr Barry GARDINER

Population million number 35

466	Hexham	86	17	21	Con	Mr Peter ATKINSON
467	Welwyn Hatfield	86	20	21	Lab	Miss Melanie JOHNSON
468	Harrow East	86	16	21	Lab	Mr Tony McNULTY
469	Wellingborough	86	18	21	Lab	Mr Paul STINCHCOMBE
470	Stourbridge	86	17	21	Lab	Ms Debra SHIPLEY
471	North Norfolk	86	17	21	Con	Mr David PRIOR
472	Sleaford and North Hykeham	86	16	21	Con	The Rt Hon Douglas HOGG
473	Leeds North West	85	20	21	Lab	Mr Harold BEST
474	Uxbridge	85	17	20	Con	Sir Michael SHERSBY
475	Congleton	85	14	20	Con	Mrs Ann WINTERTON
476	Kettering	85	16	20	Lab	Mr Philip SAWFORD
477	Bridgwater	85	17	20	Con	The Rt Hon Tom KING
478	Beckenham	85	16	20	Con	Mr Piers MERCHANT

Population million number 36

479	Skipton and Ripon	85	16	20	Con	The Rt Hon David CURRY
480	Lewes	85	16	20	Lib Dem	Mr Norman BAKER
481	Mid Worcestershire	84	16	20	Con	Mr Peter LUFF
482	Selby	84	15	20	Lab	Mr John GROGAN
483	Hendon	84	20	20	Lab	Mr Andrew DISMORE
484	Westmorland and Lonsdale	84	16	20	Con	Mr Tim COLLINS
485	Norwich North	84	19	19	Lab	Mr Ian GIBSON
486	Bath	84	20	19	Lib Dem	Mr Don FOSTER
487	Chichester	84	17	19	Con	Mr Andrew TYRIE
488	Macclesfield	84	15	19	Con	Mr Nicholas WINTERTON
489	Ashford	84	17	19	Con	Mr Damian GREEN
490	Bosworth	83	15	19	Con	Mr David TREDINNICK
491	Ruislip-Northwood	83	14	19	Con	Mr John WILKINSON

Population million number 37

492	Kingswood	83	16	19	Lab	Mr Roger BERRY
493	Epping Forest	83	15	19	Con	Mrs Eleanor LAING

494	South West Bedfordshire	83	15	19	Con	Sir David MADEL
495	Pudsey	83	17	18	Lab	Mr Paul TRUSWELL
496	Eastleigh	83	14	18	Lib Dem	David CHIDGEY
497	Gillingham	83	16	18	Lab	Mr Paul CLARK
498	Wycombe	83	15	18	Con	Sir Ray WHITNEY
499	Sutton and Cheam	83	13	18	Lib Dem	Mr Paul BURSTOW
500	Bexleyheath and Crayford	83	15	18	Lab	Mr Nigel BEARD
501	Watford	83	17	18	Lab	Miss Claire WARD
502	Aldershot	83	15	18	Con	Mr Gerald HOWARTH
503	Basingstoke	83	16	18	Con	Mr Andrew HUNTER
504	Canterbury	83	18	18	Con	Mr Julian BRAZIER

Population million number 38

505	Bromley and Chislehurst	82	15	18	Con	Mr Eric FORTH
506	Reading East	82	17	18	Lab	Ms Jane GRIFFITHS
507	Romford	82	15	18	Lab	Ms Eileen GORDON
508	New Forest East	82	13	17	Con	Dr Julian LEWIS
509	Stevenage	82	21	17	Lab	Ms Barbara FOLLETT
510	Ryedale	82	16	17	Con	John GREENWAY
511	Richmond	82	16	17	Con	The Rt Hon William HAGUE
512	Lichfield	82	14	17	Con	Mr Michael FABRICANT
513	Vale of York	81	15	17	Con	Mrs Anne McINTOSH
514	Billericay	81	16	17	Con	Mrs Teresa GORMAN
515	Monmouth	81	16	17	Lab	Mr Huw EDWARDS
516	Yeovil	81	17	17	Lib Dem	The Rt Hon Paddy ASHDOWN
517	Beverley and Holderness	81	16	17	Con	Mr James CRAN

Population million number 39

518	Hertsmere	81	15	17	Con	Mr James CLAPPISON
519	West Aberdeenshire and Kincardine	81	15	17	Lib Dem	Sir Bob SMITH
520	Maldon and East Chelmsford	81	14	17	Con	Mr John WHITTINGDALE
521	Aylesbury	81	15	16	Con	Mr David LIDINGTON
522	Broxtowe	81	16	16	Lab	Dr Nicholas PALMER
523	Redditch	81	19	16	Lab	Mrs Jacqui SMITH
524	Devizes	81	18	16	Con	The Rt Hon Michael ANCRAM
525	Westbury	81	15	16	Con	Mr David FABER
526	Newbury	81	15	16	Lib Dem	Mr David RENDEL
527	North West Cambridgeshire	81	17	16	Con	The Rt Hon Dr Brian MAWHINNEY
528	Bromsgrove	81	15	16	Con	Ms Julie KIRKBRIDE
529	South East Cornwall	81	16	16	Lib Dem	Mr Colin BREED
530	Tiverton and Honiton	81	16	16	Con	Mrs Angela BROWNING

Population million number 40

531	East Hampshire	81	13	16	Con	Mr Michael MATES
532	Broxbourne	81	14	16	Con	Mrs Marion ROE
533	Stratford on Avon	80	15	16	Con	Mr John MAPLES
534	Loughborough	80	17	16	Lab	Mr Andrew REED
535	New Forest West	80	14	15	Con	Mr Desmond SWAYNE
536	Ludlow	80	16	15	Con	Mr Christopher GILL
537	Kingston and Surbiton	80	16	15	Lib Dem	Mr Edward DAVEY
538	Maidstone and the Weald	80	15	15	Con	Miss Ann WIDDECOMBE
539	Bexhill and Battle	80	15	15	Con	Mr Charles WARDLE
540	East Surrey	80	13	15	Con	Mr Peter AINSWORTH
541	Leominster	80	15	15	Con	Mr Peter TEMPLE-MORRIS
542	West Derbyshire	79	16	15	Con	Mr Patrick McLOUGHLIN
543	Finchley and Golders Green	79	19	15	Lab	Dr Rudi VIS

Population million number 41

544	Epsom and Ewell	79	12	15	Con	The Rt Hon Sir Archie HAMILTON
545	Rushcliffe	79	14	15	Con	The Rt Hon Kenneth CLARKE
546	Sevenoaks	79	14	15	Con	Mr Michael FALLON
547	West Suffolk	79	19	14	Con	Mr Richard SPRING
548	Rutland and Melton	79	15	14	Con	Mr Alan DUNCAN
549	Chingford and Woodford Green	79	17	14	Con	Mr Iain DUNCAN-SMITH
550	St Albans	79	15	14	Lab	Mr Kerry POLLARD
551	Fareham	79	12	14	Con	The Rt Hon Sir Peter LLOYD
552	Richmond Park	78	17	14	Lib Dem	Dr Jenny TONGE
553	Harborough	78	13	14	Con	Mr Edward GARNIER
554	Castle Point	78	13	14	Lab	Ms Christine BUTLER
555	Spelthorne	78	13	14	Con	Mr David WILSHIRE
556	Banbury	78	17	13	Con	Mr Tony BALDRY

Population million number 42

557	Hemel Hempstead	78	18	13	Lab	Mr Tony McWALTER
558	Southend West	78	16	13	Con	Mr David AMESS
559	Runnymede and Weybridge	78	14	13	Con	Mr Philip HAMMOND
560	Totnes	78	17	13	Con	Mr Anthony STEEN
561	Orpington	78	14	13	Con	Mr John HORAM
562	Brentwood and Ongar	78	13	13	Con	Mr Eric PICKLES
563	Wimbledon	78	17	13	Lab	Mr Roger CASALE
564	Maidenhead	77	12	12	Con	Mrs Theresa MAY
565	East Devon	77	16	12	Con	The Rt Hon Sir Peter EMERY
566	Somerton and Frome	77	15	12	Lib Dem	Mr David HEATH
567	Twickenham	77	15	12	Lib Dem	Dr Vincent CABLE
568	North Wiltshire	77	15	12	Con	Mr James GRAY
569	Tewkesbury	77	14	12	Con	Mr Laurence ROBERTSON

Population million number 43

570	Central Suffolk and North Ipswich	77	16	12	Con	Mr Michael LORD
571	Haltemprice and Howden	77	12	12	Con	Mr David DAVIS
572	Charnwood	77	12	12	Con	The Rt Hon Stephen DORRELL
573	Faversham and Mid Kent	77	17	12	Con	Mr Andrew ROWE
574	Hitchin and Harpenden	77	14	12	Con	The Rt Hon Peter LILLEY
575	Cambridge	77	23	12	Lab	Ms Anne CAMPBELL
576	Tunbridge Wells	77	16	12	Con	Mr Archie NORMAN
577	South West Hertfordshire	77	15	12	Con	Mr Richard PAGE
578	West Worcestershire	76	15	11	Con	Sir Michael SPICER
579	North East Hertfordshire	76	17	11	Con	Mr Oliver HEALD
580	North Essex	76	13	11	Con	The Hon Bernard JENKIN
581	Wealden	76	12	11	Con	The Rt Hon Sir Geoffrey JOHNSON SMITH
582	South West Devon	76	12	11	Con	Mr Gary STREETER
583	Cotswold	76	17	11	Con	Mr Geoffrey CLIFTON-BROWN

Population million number 44

584	Bracknell	76	15	11	Con	Mr Andrew MacKAY
585	Huntingdon	76	15	11	Con	The Rt Hon John MAJOR
586	Stroud	76	15	11	Lab	Mr David DREW
587	Mid Norfolk	76	14	10	Con	Mr Keith SIMPSON
588	Southgate	76	15	10	Lab	Mr Stephen TWIGG
589	Christchurch	75	13	10	Con	Mr Christopher CHOPE
590	Hertford and Stortford	75	14	10	Con	Mr Bowen WELLS

591	Milton Keynes North East	75	16	10	Lab	Mr Brian WHITE
592	Braintree	75	18	10	Lab	Mr Alan HURST
593	Mid Dorset and North Poole	75	13	10	Con	Mr Christopher FRASER
594	Rayleigh	75	11	10	Con	Dr Michael CLARK
595	Harrow West	75	15	10	Lab	Mr Gareth THOMAS

Population million number 45

596	Wansdyke	75	13	10	Lab	Mr Dan NORRIS
597	South Staffordshire	75	13	10	Con	Sir Patrick CORMACK
598	Blaby	75	12	10	Con	Mr Andrew ROBATHAN
599	North Dorset	75	15	10	Con	Mr Robert WALTER
600	Windsor	75	14	10	Con	Hon Michael TREND
601	Old Bexley and Sidcup	75	13	9	Con	The Rt Hon Sir Edward HEATH
602	South East Cambridgeshire	75	15	9	Con	Mr James PAICE
603	Mid Bedfordshire	75	13	9	Con	Mr Jonathan SAYEED
604	Winchester	75	15	9	Lib Dem	Mr Mark OATEN
605	Croydon South	74	12	9	Con	Mr Richard OTTAWAY
606	Daventry	74	15	9	Con	Mr Tim BOSWELL
607	Sutton Coldfield	74	12	9	Con	The Rt Hon Sir Norman FOWLER
608	Chipping Barnet	74	14	9	Con	Sir Sydney CHAPMAN

Population million number 46

609	Horsham	74	13	9	Con	Rt Hon Francis MAUDE
610	Guildford	74	15	9	Con	Mr Nick ST AUBYN
611	Oxford West and Abingdon	74	16	8	Lib Dem	Dr Evan HARRIS
612	South West Surrey	74	14	8	Con	The Rt Hon Mrs Virginia BOTTOMLEY
613	Bury St Edmunds	74	16	8	Con	Mr David RUFFLEY
614	Solihull	74	12	8	Con	Mr John M. TAYLOR
615	Mid Sussex	73	13	8	Con	Hon Nicholas SOAMES
616	Surrey Heath	73	11	7	Con	Mr Nick HAWKINS
617	Mole Valley	73	13	7	Con	Sir Paul BERESFORD
618	North West Hampshire	73	16	7	Con	The Rt Hon Sir George YOUNG
619	Wantage	73	15	7	Con	Mr Robert JACKSON
620	Tonbridge and Malling	73	16	7	Con	The Rt Hon Sir John STANLEY

Population million (remainder) number 47*

621	Suffolk Coastal	72	16	6	Con	The Rt Hon John GUMMER
622	Arundel and South Downs	72	13	6	Con	Mr Howard FLIGHT
623	Beaconsfield	72	12	6	Con	Mr Dominic GRIEVE
624	Woking	72	14	6	Con	Mr Humfrey MALINS
625	Cheadle	71	11	5	Con	Mr Stephen DAY
626	North East Hampshire	71	12	5	Con	Mr James ARBUTHNOT
627	Henley	71	13	5	Con	The Rt Hon Michael HESELTINE
628	Saffron Walden	71	14	4	Con	Sir Alan HASELHURST

'Best health' million

629	Buckingham	71	13	4	Con	Mr John BERCOW
630	Northavon	70	11	3	Lib Dem	Prof Steve WEBB
631	Esher and Walton	69	13	2	Con	Mr Ian TAYLOR
632	Witney	69	15	2	Con	Mr Shaun WOODWARD
633	South Suffolk	69	15	2	Con	Mr Tim YEO
634	West Chelmsford	69	15	2	Con	Mr Simon BURNS
635	South Norfolk	69	14	1	Con	The Rt Hon John MacGREGOR
636	Chesham and Amersham	67	11	0	Con	Mrs Cheryl GILLAN
637	South Cambridgeshire	66	14	-2†	Con	Mr Andrew LANSLEY

638	Sheffield Hallam	66	15	-2†	Lib Dem	Mr Richard ALLAN
639	Romsey	65	12	-5†	Con	Mr Michael COLVIN
640	Woodspring	65	12	-5†	Con	Dr Liam FOX
641	Wokingham	65	10	-5†	Con	The Rt Hon John REDWOOD

Note: * As the total population of Britain under the age of 65 totals 47,587,310 this groups contains less than one million people aged under 65.

†Avoidable deaths are negative for the lowest mortality constituencies in the 'best health' million – as they have better than average mortality for that privileged group as a whole.

Appendix B: Technical details for estimating numbers living in poverty

It is possible to estimate the numbers of poor children and poor households at the community level (using the *Breadline Britain* definitions of poverty; see Gordon and Pantazis, 1997) by obtaining weightings for the best subset of deprivation indicator variables that were measured in both the 1991 Census and the *Breadline Britain* survey and by then using the multivariate statistical technique of logistic regression (Gordon and Forrest, 1995; Gordon, 1995).

Eleven variables, which have been used in one or more Census-based indices, were examined to estimate the number living in poverty.

V1   Unemployment
V2   Lone parents
V3   Limiting long-term illness
V4   Low social class
V5   No access to a car
V6   Living in non-owner-occupier accommodation
V7   Single pensioners
V8   Divorced people
V9   Widows
V10   Lacking or sharing basic amenities
V11   Not self-contained accommodation

A step-wise logistic regression analysis allowed the best subset of variables to be selected that were proxies of poverty (as defined by the *Breadline Britain* survey) and provided weightings for each variable after allowing for the overlaps between variables (ie lone-parent households may also be likely to be of low social class or live in rented accommodation).

There was a considerable degree of overlap between single pensioners and widows and both variables were excluded because they were not good predictors of poverty. Divorced people were excluded because of their high overlap with single parenthood, which was a better predictor of poverty. 'Lacking basic amenities' and 'not self-contained accommodation' were dropped because they were found not to be additive, for example, households which contained someone with a limiting long-term illness and also lacked basic amenities were not likely to be poorer than a household with an ill person but with basic amenities. The reason for this is that many poor disabled people live in local authority accommodation which invariably have indoor toilets and bathrooms.

An estimate of the number of poor households in an area can be calculated as: 21.7% of the number of households with no access to a car + 20.3% of the number of households not in owner-occupied accommodation + 16% of the number of lone-parent households + 15.9% of the number of workers in social classes IV and V + 10.8% of the number of households containing a person with a limiting long-term illness + 9.4% of unemployed workers.

The evidence presented in Chapter 2 demonstrated that there is a clear causal relationship between poverty and ill-health, and this is taken up again in Chapter 4. Figure B1 shows a scatter plot of the estimated percentage of poor households (calculated using the *Breadline Britain* method described above) against the Standardised Illness Ratio (SIR) for the 8,519 electoral wards of England, calculated from the Limiting Long-Term Illness question in the 1991 Census. The regression line with a 95% Confidence Interval is also shown. There appears to be very good agreement between these two variables (Pearson's Product Moment Correlation 0.82).

Figure B1: Poor households by Standardised Illness Ratio (SIR) in England (1991)

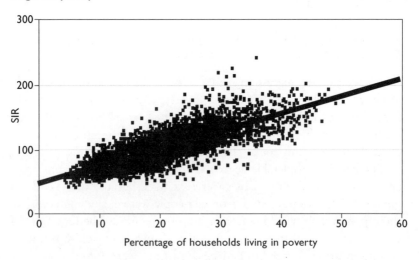

Source: Analysis by authors

Because of concerns that the inclusion of LLTI led to circular reasoning (ie that the poverty index predicted mortality because our poverty indicator included a measure of morbidity) the above procedure was repeated, but omitting LLTI. The result was only a slight adjustment of the regression parameters and the inclusion of the proportion of households having or sharing use of bath/shower and/or inside WC (ie basic amenities).

This amended estimate of the number of poor households was calculated as: 27.2% of the number of households in not in owner-occupied accommodation + 18.8% of the number of households with no access to a car + 26.5% of the number of lone-parent households + 19.6% of the number of workers in social classes IV and V + 17.1% of unemployed workers + 17.9% of households lacking basic amenities.

This amended poverty indicator was compared to that including LLTI as a predictor and the two were found to be almost interchangeable, as Figure B2 shows. We have therefore used the original indicator throughout. Part of the reason for using this original version is the argument about the lacking basic amenities variables, discussed above.

Figure B2: **Scatterplot of original poverty indicator (with LLTI) and the amended poverty indicator (without LLTI), constituencies in Britain (1991)**

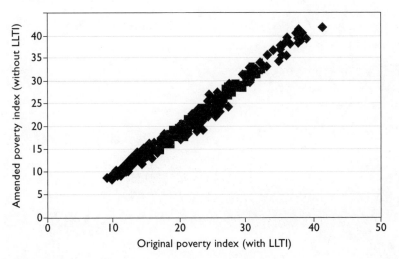

Source: Analysis by authors

Appendix C: Does the spatial distribution of social class explain geographical inequalities in health?

It would be easy to assume that the compositional effect of differential social class distributions between areas explains a large part of the geographical inequality in mortality between areas. Unfortunately a breakdown of class by age is only available from Sample of Anonymised Records (SAR) areas (see Dale and Marsh, 1993) and age/class specific mortality ratios are only available from the Longitudinal Study of England and Wales. Nevertheless we can use these sources to test the importance of class distribution by applying the age-class specific mortality rates by social class to the numbers of people living in each SAR area to determine the expected mortality in an area having allowed for both age and social class structure. Here we do this for men only as mortality rates by both age and class have not recently been published for women.

Table C1 gives age-class specific mortality rates for men in Britain calculated from the 1% Longitudinal Study sample. The 2% Sample of Anonymised Areas from the 1991 Census provides an estimate of the numbers of men of these ages and classes for 253 areas in England and Wales. Given these two data sources and an estimate of what fraction of the actual population are represented by the SAR it is simple to calculate how many men of these ages we would expect to have died in any of the 253 SAR areas. These age-class standardised mortality ratios can then be compared to simple age standardised ratios to estimate the extent to which variations in the spatial distribution of social classes can explain the spatial variations in mortality in Britain.

Table C1: **Age-specific mortality rate by social class, all causes, England and Wales (1991-93)**

Men	25-29	30-34	35-39	40-44	45-49	50-54	55-59	60-64
I	91	142	228	373	704	1,186	2,057	3,735
II	146	197	279	380	722	1,230	2,148	3,992
IIINM	181	319	448	600	1,125	1,773	2,975	5,414
IIIM	221	279	429	619	1,141	1,989	3,521	6,736
IV	260	325	485	681	1,244	2,020	3,491	6,227
V	489	660	950	1,334	2,047	3,430	5,534	9,341
All others	246	250	307	425	579	1,035	1,745	2,996

Note: Remainder line for all others uses average rates for all men of these ages.
Source: Drever and Bunting (1997, Table 8.3)

To illustrate our method, the total numbers of men by class in the SAR are shown in Table C2 for the SAR area of the 1991 Manchester district. Excluding Scotland, Manchester contains the greatest concentration of people living in the worst off areas in Britain referred to in this book. The total population figures are taken from the 'Estimating with Confidence Project', which adjusts the census to allow for people who were not included in the 1991 Census (Simpson and Dorling, 1994). The SAR undersamples men due to its sampling strategy as a representative household (rather than individual) sample and due to Census underenumeration.

Table C2: **2% sample of the male population by social class and age in Manchester (1991)**

Men	25-29	30-34	35-39	40-44	45-49	50-54	55-59	60-64	Total
I	30	25	24	13	6	9	5	4	116
II	74	63	60	45	33	18	20	24	337
IIINM	33	29	21	17	10	11	15	17	153
IIIM	80	77	72	70	58	54	56	49	516
IV	49	40	24	26	27	33	35	33	267
V	24	26	21	10	13	15	13	12	134
All others	8	7	5	5	3	1	5	3	37
Total	298	267	227	186	150	141	149	142	1,560
1991 population	22,406	16,139	12,341	12,134	9,689	9,463	9,599	9,615	101,386
Sampling	67%	83%	92%	77%	77%	75%	78%	74%	77%

Note: The sampling fractions are the proportion of a perfect 2% sample (as the SAR is a household sample).
Source: Analysis by authors

If the matrix of population for Manchester is multiplied through by the national matrix of mortality rates, adjusted to allow for sampling fractions, then the estimated number of men to have died in the three-year period 1990 to 1992 is as shown in Table C3 below.

Table C3: **Estimate of male deaths by social class and age in Manchester (1990-92)**

Men	25-29	30-34	35-39	40-44	45-49	50-54	55-59	60-64	Total
I	2	2	3	3	3	7	7	10	37
II	8	8	9	11	15	15	28	65	159
IIINM	4	6	5	7	7	13	29	62	133
IIIM	13	13	17	28	43	72	127	223	537
IV	10	8	6	12	22	45	79	139	320
V	9	10	11	9	17	35	46	76	213
All others	1	1	1	11	1	6	6	18	
Total	48	48	52	71	108	187	321	582	1,416

Source: Tables C1 and C2

Between 1990 and 1992, 2,063 men died between the ages of 25 and 64 in Manchester. Given national age-specific mortality rates we would have expected 1,294 to have died, giving an area SMR for this age and sex group of 159. Taking into account variations in the class structure of Manchester increases the numbers of deaths expected to 1,416 and reduces the mortality ratio to 146, thus accounting for a sixth of the excess mortality in that city. For England and Wales, the inclusion of social class reduces the numbers of excess deaths by area per year by only 29%.

Index